WABI SABI

Also by Beth Kempton

Freedom Seeker:
Live More. Worry Less. Do What You Love.

BETH KEMPTON

WABI SABI

JAPANESE WISDOM
FOR A PERFECTLY
IMPERFECT LIFE

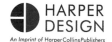

HARPER
DESIGN
An Imprint of HarperCollins Publishers

First published in Great Britain in 2018 by Piatkus.
Wabi Sabi

HarperCollins books may be purchased for educational,
business, or sales promotional use. For information please email
the Special Markets Department at SPsales@harpercollins.com.

Published in 2019 by
Harper Design
An Imprint of HarperCollins*Publishers*
195 Broadway
New York, NY 10007
Tel: (212) 207-7000
Fax: (855) 746-6023
harperdesign@harpercollins.com
www.hc.com

Distributed throughout the world by
HarperCollins Publishers
195 Broadway
New York, NY 10007

ISBN 978-0-06-290515-4

Library of Congress Control Number 2018955232

Printed in Italy

Fifth Printing, 2021

To my family.
I love you just the way you are.

A note on the use of Japanese in this book

Japanese personal names have been written in standard English name order for ease of reference (first name followed by surname), except for historical figures most commonly known by the traditional Japanese name order (family name first), such as Matsuo Bashō (family name of Matsuo).

The modified Hepburn system has been used to romanize the Japanese language. Macrons have been used to indicate long vowels; for example, *ū* for an extended *uu*. This includes place names, even if they are familiarly known without the macrons, such as Tōkyō and Kyōto.

When referencing people, the suffix *-san* is sometimes used. This is a polite way to say "Mr.," "Mrs.," or "Ms." When the suffix *-sensei* is used, this refers to a teacher or professor.

CONTENTS

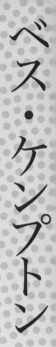

ベス・ケンプトン

ABOUT
THE AUTHOR

Beth Kempton has been inhaling the magic and mystery of Japan and has been influenced by its philosophy and aesthetics for more than two decades. With a master's degree in Japanese, Beth has spent many years living and working in Japan, which she considers her second home. Over the years, she has taken lessons in Japanese papermaking, flower arranging, pottery, *noren*-making, calligraphy, tea ceremony practice, and weaving. Collectively, these experiences have led to a deep love of the country and a rare understanding of cultural and linguistic nuances.

Beth previously trained in television presenter skills at NTV in Tōkyō and, many moons ago, hosted her own show on Yamagata Cable Television in the north of the country. She has written about Japan and Oriental philosophy in various publications including *Wanderlust, Yoga Magazine,* and *Where Women Create.*

Beth is also an award-winning entrepreneur and self-help author, and cofounder of the online design magazine *MOYŌ* (which is Japanese for "pattern"). Together with her husband, Mr. K, she runs dowhatyouloveforlife.com, makeartthatsells.com, and makeitindesign.com—all of which offer tools, resources, and online courses for living an inspired life. Beth also coleads an online members' club for soulful women entrepreneurs at hellosoulhellobusiness.com, and mentors individuals through times of major life and career change (see bethkempton.com for details).

Named a "Rising Star" by *Spirit & Destiny* magazine, Beth was also nominated *Kindred Spirit* magazine Mind Body Spirit Blogger of the Year 2017, and her blog was recently named one of the best happiness blogs on the planet. Her first book, *Freedom Seeker: Live More. Worry Less. Do What You Love.*, was published by Hay House in 2017. She loves leading workshops and speaking live, and is on the faculty of 1440 Multiversity in California.

Beth describes herself as a wanderer, an adventurer, and a seeker of beauty, with a slight obsession with chocolate and Japanese stationery. The mother of two adorable girls, she lives a slow-ish life on the south coast of England, and loves nothing more than a dose of *shinrin-yoku* (forest bathing) and a picnic with her young family. You can take a peek at her perfectly imperfect life on Instagram @bethkempton.

Find Beth here:
www.bethkempton.com
www.dowhatyouloveforlife.com
www.facebook.com/dowhatyoulovexx
Instagram @bethkempton
Twitter @dowhatyoulovexx
Podcast: www.bethkempton.com/podcast

前書き

At the age of twenty-one, I left Japan to make my way in the big, wide world. The eight years I spent playing in the Italian League Serie A and the English Premier League were, as a professional footballer, the most important in my athletic career. As a person, the experience of living abroad showed me how stepping outside the familiar can really open our eyes and minds.

During those years, I worked hard to learn first Italian and then English. The more I learned, the more I discovered how language offers a window into other cultures, and can be a doorway to lifelong friendships.

After retiring from football following the 2006 FIFA World Cup, I spent the next few years traveling all over the world, meeting people from all walks of life. Everywhere I went, people would tell me that they were interested in Japan. They asked me all sorts of questions, many of which I could not answer. And I realized then, that even though I was Japanese, there was a depth and richness to my own culture that I had not yet truly appreciated. I wanted to understand what it was that was so appealing to people worldwide, so I made the decision to go back to Japan and find out for myself.

I carried with me the question "What is culture?" Food culture, fashion culture, Japanese culture . . . I wanted to understand this idea more. When people use the term "culture" they refer to a certain lifestyle followed by a number of people over a period of time—something we create by the way we live. So I decided to visit people instead of places.

I spent the next seven years exploring every corner of Japan, visiting all of the forty-seven prefectures to spend time with artisans, farmers, sake brewers, Zen monks, Shintō priests, and local people. And while I set out to learn about Japanese culture, I ended up learning about life.

Every time I woke before the sun to spend time with farmers harvesting their rice, smelled the air before the rains came, or watched craftsmen coax beauty from materials that grew in their shadow, I learned what it means to live in harmony with the earth. The juicy fruit, just picked from the vine, the freshly caught fish, the carefully brewed sake—with each bite and sip I learned more about how to really taste.

As time went on, I noticed I was falling into the rhythm of country life, which is the rhythm of the seasons and of nature in Japan. Living in cities, we have access to so many good things, but, at the same time, we are separated from nature and the artificial environment can sap our energy. It was only when I spent month after month in the countryside that I realized how much better I felt. More energized, alert, and happy.

When we separate ourselves from nature it becomes something we attempt to manage and control. But it can release its awesome power at any moment. I believe it's when we live in relationship with nature, respecting it and flowing in rhythm with it, that we feel at our best and appreciate each day, moment by moment.

Wabi sabi is intimately intertwined with this fundamental relationship with nature. It relates to the acceptance of the transience of all things, and the experiencing of life with all the senses. I hope this book inspires you to find your own gentle rhythm and discover happiness right where you are.

Having known Beth for more than twelve years, and knowing her commitment as a student of Japanese life, I know she is the one to take you on this journey.

Hidetoshi Nakata
Tōkyō, 2018

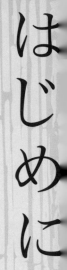

はじめに

INTRODUCTION

t is a cold December night in Kyōto, the ancient capital of Japan. I have cycled through the darkness to Shōren-in, a small temple off the tourist trail, that is nestled at the foot of the Higashiyama mountains. Tonight, the temple gardens are gently illuminated, the low light spinning a mysterious yarn across the silhouetted pines and chimerical bamboo groves.

I remove my shoes and step inside, onto a floor polished to a high shine by eight hundred years of shuffling footsteps and swishing robes. The wide floorboards, mottled and darkened with age, hail from the Imperial Palace. I take a seat on the wraparound veranda at the back, my toes numb from the cold and my breath visible in front of my face.

Incense fills the air. It smells like the color purple, in a way I cannot explain. Tiny lights scattered across the garden fade in and out, a thousand stars breathing in unison. Just ten minutes away, the entertainment district of Gion is bustling with the energy of excitable tourists, drunken businessmen, and attentive geisha. But here, up a narrow, sloping road on the eastern edge of the city, I have found stillness.

Overhead, a chenille moon is peeping through the trees, casting its silvery spell across the pond. Fallen leaves skate over the surface, as koi skulk through the milky waters below. A week from now the branches of many of these trees will be bare. A month later, perhaps cloaked in snow.

I pick up a fallen momiji (maple) leaf, blushing burgundy and curling at the edges. It's a treasure, crinkled and papery, like the back of my grandmother's hand. A space in my heart opens up. Right now, I have *everything I need. I feel quiet contentment, tinged with melancholy in the knowledge that this fleeting moment will never return.*

This is the world of wabi sabi.

Discovering *wabi sabi*

Wabi sabi is fundamental to the aesthetic sense and gentle nature of the Japanese people. It is a worldview that guides the way they experience life, although it is rarely discussed. Its influence is everywhere, and yet it is nowhere to be seen. People instinctively know what the concept of *wabi sabi* represents, but few can articulate it. *Wabi sabi* is a fascinating enigma, which promises to whisper potent wisdom to those who slow down enough to investigate and approach with an open heart.

I have been visiting Japan for more than two decades and lived there for almost a third of that time. The affinity I have always felt with Japanese people belies my upbringing on the other side of the world. I have immersed myself in the culture, lived with Japanese families who speak no English, worked in the complex worlds of Japanese business and local government, spent way more than ten thousand hours studying, and traveled widely throughout the land. And yet, despite all this, a true definition of the soulful concept of *wabi sabi* has remained elusive. I could sense it but lacked the words to explain it.

A number of other non-Japanese have delved into the world of *wabi sabi* before me, and most have focused on the physical characteristics of objects and environments they associate with the idea. However, those explanations have always fallen short for me. I have long had a sense that *wabi sabi* goes much deeper than we have been led to believe, flowing into many areas of life. It wasn't until I started to research this book that I realized just how deep that river runs.

Why *wabi sabi*?

In recent years, society has gathered pace, our stress levels have gone through the roof, and we have become increasingly obsessed with money, job titles, appearances, and the endless accumulation of stuff. There is a growing sense of discontent as we push ourselves harder and juggle more. We are overworked, overstretched, and overwhelmed.

As someone who has spent the best part of a decade helping people realign their priorities to build a life focused on doing what they love, I have seen how so many of us are making ourselves ill with overcommitment, constant comparison, judgment, and negative self-talk. We are sleepwalking through our days, senses dulled, spending much of our time cooped up in boxes, paying more attention to celebrities, advertising, and social media than to the exploration of our own lives, in all their rich potential.

For some time now, I have been hearing the growing rumblings of a slow revolution, a yearning for a simpler, more meaningful life. A life infused with beauty, connected to nature, thrumming with the energy of everyday well-being, and built around what really matters to us. The more people who came to me exhausted, stuck, and unhappy, the more I felt the need for a new way to approach challenges and for accessible tools to help us live more authentic and inspired lives.

This brought to mind the underlying grace, calm, and sense of appreciation in Japan that I haven't experienced anywhere else, hinting at life lessons tucked into the sleeves of the cultural kimono. I suspected it may have something to do with the elusive concept of *wabi sabi*, so I set out to discover the hidden truth.

Defining the indefinable

As I've said, trying to articulate a definition of *wabi sabi* is a tricky endeavor. It's a bit like love—I can tell you what I think it is and how it feels to me, but it's only when you feel it for yourself that you really know. Almost without exception, conversations I have had with Japanese people on this topic have begun with: "*Wabi sabi*? Hmmm . . . It's very difficult to explain." And the truth is, most people have never tried to articulate it and don't see the need to do so. They have grown up with it. It's how they navigate the world and appreciate beauty. It is built into who they are.

However, never one to shrink from a challenge, I pressed on. Well, actually, I waited, I watched, and I listened. The more space I gave people to explore the meaning of this unspoken thing that was so familiar to them, the more interesting it became. There were metaphors and hand gestures and head tilts. There were hands on hearts and long pauses and repeated references to tea and Zen and nature. The conversation nearly always ended with: "I want to read your book."

The fact is, there is no universal definition of *wabi sabi* in the Japanese language. Any attempt to express it will only ever be from the perspective of the person explaining it.

My own perspective is that of someone in the unusual position of being both a Japanologist and a life coach. In my attempt to distill the principles of *wabi sabi* into a series of accessible life lessons, I have talked to people from all walks of life, pored over books in old libraries, visited museums, meditated in shadowy temples, held tea bowls in my hands, spent time in nature, and wandered through centuries-old Japanese architecture. After hundreds of conversations and extensive research, I have crafted a set of guiding principles that I hope will be valuable lessons for us all. You can find them all within this book.

The *wabi sabi* secret

In slowly peeling back the layers of mystery, this is what I have come to understand: the true beauty of *wabi sabi* lies not in things but in the very nature of life itself.

> *Wabi sabi* is an intuitive response to beauty that reflects the true nature of life.
>
> *Wabi sabi* is an acceptance and appreciation of the impermanent, imperfect, and incomplete nature of everything.
>
> *Wabi sabi* is a recognition of the gifts of simple, slow, and natural living.

Wabi sabi is a state of the heart. It is a deep in-breath and a slow exhale. It is felt in a moment of real appreciation—a perfect moment in an imperfect world. We can nurture it with our willingness to notice details and cultivate delight. And we experience it when we are living the most authentic, most inspired versions of our lives.

It's about experiencing the world by truly being in it rather than judging it from the sidelines. It's about allowing strategy to give way to sensitivity. It's about taking the time to pay attention.

The principles that underlie *wabi sabi* can teach us life lessons about letting go of perfection and accepting ourselves just as we are. They give us tools for escaping the chaos and material pressures of modern life, so we can be content with less. And they remind us to look for beauty in the everyday, allowing ourselves to be moved by it and, in doing so, feeling gratitude for life itself.

How to use this book

In order to understand the depth and richness of *wabi sabi*, we begin with a short history lesson that sets the scene for all that is to come. While this book is not a detailed discourse on Japanese aesthetics, history, culture, philosophy, or religion, these are all touched on to the extent that they are important threads in the fabric of Japanese life. For further reading or inspiration for your own journey of discovery, please see the bibliography (page 220) and notes on visiting Japan (page 214).

The secret of *wabi sabi* lies in seeing the world not with the logical mind but through the feeling heart.

Once we have a sense of the origins of *wabi sabi*, we will explore its characteristics, to give us language to think and talk about it. Then we will look at why this ancient wisdom is so very relevant to our lives today. All of this is covered in chapter 1, and I encourage you to read it first.

From chapter 2 onward, I share stories, inspiration, and advice for applying the concept to every area of your life. You might want to read these in order or dip in and out, depending on what calls to you most right now. There is, of course, no perfect way to read this book. It is for you to take from it what you need.

Travel with me

This book is an invitation to travel with me as a curious explorer in a foreign land. Know that you are safe with me by your side. The map I have sketched out will guide us off the beaten track, down crooked paths, through old wooden gates, into ancient forests, along winding rivers, and deep into the mountains.

Now and then, we will stop at a roadside teahouse to rest awhile and ponder, hitch lifts from strangers, and be blessed with unexpected wisdom from new friends. There will be times when we sing as we walk and times when we feel weary. We might pause to soak our aching bodies in a hot spring or be hushed by falling snow. Some days we will rise with the sun, others we will amble beneath the stars.

This book is an invitation to relax into the beauty of your life at any given moment, and to strip away all that is unnecessary, to discover what lies within.

Along the way, you'll encounter the familiar and the unknown, the old and the new. Some things will challenge the very foundations of what you have been led to believe. I'll be here with you every step of the way.

Let's commit to traveling slowly, exploring far, and going deep, as I share this ancient Japanese wisdom with you.

A search for *wabi sabi* is a journey to the heart of life itself. Open your eyes and embrace the mystery of all that is to come.

Beth Kempton
Kyōto, 2018

「侘び寂び」とは

CHAPTER 1:
ORIGINS,
CHARACTERISTICS,
AND RELEVANCE OF
WABI SABI TODAY

You could spend a lifetime in the company of Japanese people and never hear the words *wabi sabi* spoken out loud. If you open *Kōjien*, the most authoritative Japanese dictionary available today, *wabi sabi* is nowhere to be found.[1] There are long entries for the individual words *wabi* and *sabi*, but none for the combined term. It does exist in the spoken language, and there are a small number of books in Japanese about it, but generally, it lives in hearts and minds rather than on paper. I can't even remember when I first came across it. It's as if I internalized the philosophy of *wabi sabi* by osmosis during my time in Japan.

If you ask a Japanese person to explain *wabi sabi*, they will most likely recognize it but will, as I've said, struggle to formulate a definition. It's not that they don't understand it; it's that the understanding is intuitive, and this is a reflection of a very different way of thinking and learning. Outside of rote academic learning, much of what the Japanese people absorb is by watching and experiencing. For a logical, rational-thinking Westerner, this can be challenging to grasp. We want step-by-steps, how-tos, and exact translations. But offering specificity and complete explanations is not the way in Japan. To truly appreciate the wisdom in this culture, we need to be aware that it is often within the unsaid that the true message lies.

Origins of *wabi sabi*

Wabi sabi (which can be written 侘寂 or 侘び寂び)[2] originated as two separate words, both steeped in aesthetic value, with roots in literature, culture, and religion. *Wabi* is about finding beauty in simplicity, and a spiritual richness and serenity in detaching from the material world. *Sabi* is more concerned with the passage of time, with the way that all things grow and decay and how aging alters the visual nature of those things.

It's less about *what* we see and more about *how* we see.

Both concepts are important in Japanese culture, but perhaps even more fascinating is the meaning they take on when combined to become *wabi sabi*.

The setting

Imagine, if you will, the world in the mid-sixteenth century—a time of great exploration by seafaring Europeans, with the Spanish and Portuguese opening up worldwide trade routes. It was a time of colonialism and mercantilism, when many countries had national economic policies to accumulate as much gold and silver as possible.

The paint hadn't long dried on Leonardo da Vinci's *Mona Lisa*, and *David* had only emerged from Michelangelo's block of marble a few decades previously, at the turn of the century. Over in England, Shakespeare was penning his latest masterpiece.

China was flourishing under the Ming dynasty, and was way more technologically advanced than the West. It was also very cultured, with rumors that Chinese government officials were encouraged to compose poetry and practice calligraphy between official meetings.

Meanwhile, late-medieval Japan was caught up in a century of warfare and destruction. Frequent famines, fires, and natural disasters plagued the nation, taxation was high and poverty widespread. Society was so torn apart that many ordinary folk sought solace in Buddhism, which was having a significant influence on the way people lived.

An emperor and a court were in place, but the shōgun (military leader) had the true power. The country was ruled by a class of military feudal lords known as *daimyō*, who established local territorial domains, wielded their power from newly built castles, and installed samurai warriors in the towns around those castles to protect them and serve in their armies.

The higher-ranking samurai were well educated and powerful, and known for their extreme loyalty and dedication to the service of their *daimyō* lord. Zen Buddhism was popular among them, due to its emphasis on discipline and meditation. A number of the great temples of the capital, Kyōto, were home to *karesansui* (dry-landscape gardens), said to reflect the essence of nature and inspire deep contemplation.

Many samurai had developed an interest in the ritual of tea, both because of the physical boost—it helped them to stay awake on long watches—and the spiritual benefit of creating moments of peace and harmony in their violent lives. They lived ready to die, so they welcomed opportunities to appreciate beauty in a life that could be over at any moment.

It was a time of growth for major urban areas, and Japan was seeing the rise of the merchant class. They were making a fortune as moneylenders to samurai, who were permitted to earn only a capped stipend. This industry was on the edge of the law, so merchants risked having their riches taken away at any time, meaning that they, too, were motivated to enjoy it while it lasted.

As a result, although many ordinary people were still living in relative poverty, the ruling and merchant classes had a tendency for lavish spending. Ornate castles boasted screens embellished with gold. Extravagant social events were popular among the wealthy, particularly tea gatherings. Those in power had a penchant for Chinese tea bowls and utensils, and these were rapidly becoming status symbols. An astute observer might have sensed the emergence of conflicting ideas of tea as a spiritual experience and tea-utensil collecting as a showy demonstration of wealth.

Now, hold that thought as we take a quick detour into the history of tea.

The tea connection

To explore the origin of the word *wabi* we must venture into the world of tea. The powdered green *matcha* tea now associated with the tea ceremony didn't arrive in Japan until 1191. It was brought back from China during the Song dynasty by the monk Myōan Eisai, who is credited with founding the Rinzai school of Zen Buddhism in Japan. Tea seeds were planted in three places, including Uji near Kyōto, which would remain a world-class tea producer for centuries to come. Zen, and the tea ideal, spread rapidly during this time.

As far back as the fifteenth century, monk and tea master Murata Shukō had recognized that the act of preparing and drinking tea could be a reflection of Zen principles, and as a result he is credited with a founding role in the development of the tea ceremony. Shōgun Yoshimasa, an advocate of cultural pastimes, commissioned a bespoke tea ceremony from Shukō,[3] who used this opportunity to take tea to a deeper level. According to Okakura Kakuzo in his seminal essay, *The Book of Tea*, Japan would soon raise the cult of "Teaism" into "a religion of aestheticism … founded on the adoration of the beautiful among the sordid facts of everyday existence."[4]

This simplification was taken a step further by a man named Takeno Jōō, who studied under two of Shukō's disciples in the first half of the sixteenth century. Jōō was a poet, with a talent for expressing tea ideals in verse. He made changes to the tearoom to include materials in their natural state, and would later be an important influence for Sen no Rikyū, a businessman and tea master for Toyotomi Hideyoshi, one of Japan's most famous warlords.

In time, Sen no Rikyū would become known as the true father of tea.

Simplicity as an aesthetic ideal

By the second half of the sixteenth century, the tea ceremony had become an important social event and an opportunity for the rich to display their wealth. Hideyoshi filled his ostentatious all-gold teahouse with expensive paraphernalia, mostly imported from China. At the same time, his own tea master, Sen no Rikyū, was quietly starting a revolution, reducing the physical space of the tearoom significantly to alter the fundamental principles of related aesthetic ideals, stripping everything back to what was really necessary: a space to gather, a nod to nature, a kettle, and basic implements—and time for tea.

At little over ten square feet, Sen no Rikyū's intimate tearoom was less than half the traditional size. The tiny windows reduced the light level to a minimum, so that guests had a heightened experience of their other senses. The host and guests were positioned so close together that they could hear one another breathing.

Rikyū replaced an expensive celadon vase with a bamboo flower container, and a costly Chinese bowl with one fashioned by a tile maker by the name of Chōjirō.[5] He used a bamboo tea scoop instead of an ivory one and upcycled a humble well bucket in place of an extravagant bronze water container.

Rikyū also made the significant move of bringing in all the utensils at the beginning of the ceremony and removing them all at the end. This kept the room clear and simple, allowing the guests to settle their attention on the act of making tea, the delicate natural beauty of the carefully chosen seasonal flowers, and the thought-provoking poetic calligraphy in the alcove. It was all about the shared experience, in that particular moment.

In one fell swoop, Rikyū changed the culture of tea from worshipping wealth to worshipping simplicity. And the contrast with Hideyoshi's aesthetic choices could not have been more stark. It was a bold and radical step away from tradition and the general view of what was desirable. In a time of austerity among the masses, Rikyū railed against the prevailing culture of excess in the ruling classes, bringing aesthetics back to basics: to the simple, ascetic beauty that inspired reflection on the nature of life itself.

The origins of *wabi*

Although Rikyū did not invent the tea ceremony, in the last years of his life he brought it back to the philosophy of simplicity and natural beauty that remains important in Japanese culture today. Rikyū's tea came to be known as "*wabi* tea."

The word *wabi* (which can be written 侘 or 侘び) means "subdued taste."[6] It originally had linguistic connections to poverty, insufficiency, and despair, from the verb *wabiru* (侘びる—to worry or pine)[7] and the related adjective *wabishii* (侘びしい—wretched, lonely, poor).[8]

As such, it was reflected in Japanese literature many centuries before Rikyū's time—for example, in the eighth-century *Man'yōshū* (*The Collection of Ten Thousand Leaves*), the oldest existing collection of Japanese poetry, in Kamo no Chōmei's famous short work "Hōjōki" ("An Account of My Hut"), written in 1212, and in the poetry of Fujiwara no Teika (1162–1241).[9] But it was with Rikyū's tea ceremony that *wabi* came to represent the aesthetic value of simplicity.

As an aesthetic term, the beauty of *wabi* is in its underlying tone of darkness. It is sublime beauty among the harsh realities of life. As Buddhist priest Kenkō wrote, seven centuries ago, "Should we look at the spring blossoms only in full flower, or the moon only when cloudless and clear?"[10] Beauty is not only evident in the joyous, the loud, or the obvious.

Wabi implies a stillness, with an air of rising above the mundane. It is an acceptance of reality and the insight that comes with that. It allows us to realize that whatever our situation, there is beauty hiding somewhere.

Wabi can describe the feeling generated by recognizing the beauty found in simplicity. It is a sense of quiet contentment found away from the trappings of a materialistic world. Over the years, tastes have changed and there are many decorative tea utensils available these days, but the *wabi* ideal remains part of the philosophy of tea in Japan.

Ultimately, *wabi* is a mind-set that appreciates humility, simplicity, and frugality as routes to tranquility and contentment. The spirit of *wabi* is deeply connected to the idea of accepting that our true needs are simple, and of being humble and grateful for the beauty that already exists right where we are.

The origins of *sabi*

The word *sabi* (which can be written 寂 or 寂び) means "patina, antique look, elegant simplicity."[11] The same character can also translate as "tranquility."[12] The adjective *sabishii* (寂しい) means "lonely," "lonesome," or "solitary."[13] The essence of *sabi* permeated much of Matsuo Bashō's haiku, penned in the seventeenth century and still loved all over the world for its haunting beauty.

There also exists a verb—*sabiru* (錆びる)—with a different logograph but the same reading. It means to rust, decay, or show signs of age, adding another layer of flavor.

Over time, the word *sabi* has come to communicate a deep and tranquil beauty that emerges with the passage of time. Visually, we recognize this as the patina of age, weathering, tarnishing, and signs of antiquity.

Sabi is a condition created by time, not the human hand, although it often emerges on quality objects that were originally crafted with care. It is interested in the refined elegance of age. It is beauty revealed in the processes of use and decay, such as the dull shine in the worn grain of a well-loved farmhouse kitchen table.

In his thought-provoking classic, *In Praise of Shadows*, celebrated author Jun'ichirō Tanizaki noted how Japanese people find beauty in *sabi* saying:

> We do not dislike everything that shines, but we do prefer a pensive lustre to a shallow brilliance, a murky light that, whether in a stone or an artefact, bespeaks a sheen of antiquity. . . . We do love things that bear the marks of grime, soot, and weather, and we love the colours and the sheen that call to mind the past that made them.[14]

Although *sabi* is concerned with how the passage of time manifests itself physically in objects, as with so much of Japanese aesthetics, its deeper meaning hints at what is hidden beneath the surface of the actual item that we see. It is a representation of the way all things evolve and perish and can evoke an emotional response in us, often tinged with sadness, as we reflect on the evanescence of life.

Sabi beauty reminds us of our own connection with the past, of the natural cycle of life, and of our very own mortality.

The birth of *wabi sabi*

It is a *wabi* heart that recognizes *sabi* beauty, and the two have gone hand in hand for many generations.[15] The essence of their teaching stretches back through the centuries, but the conjoined term *wabi sabi* has only emerged as a recognized term within the past hundred years or so, "as a result of a desire to understand what lies beneath the psychology of Japanese people."[16] A label was needed for what people had always known.

Wabi sabi simultaneously lives on the edge of people's consciousness and deep in their hearts. My friend Setsuko, now in her seventies, said she had never uttered *wabi sabi* out loud until I asked her about it, even though it is part of the essence of who she is, and she has an immediate sense of what it means to her.

Wabi sabi goes beyond the beauty of any given object or environment, to refer to one's response to that profound beauty. *Wabi sabi* is a feeling, and it is intangible. One person's *wabi sabi* is not the same as another's, because each of us experiences the world in different ways. We feel *wabi sabi* when we come into contact with the essence of authentic beauty—the kind that is unpretentious, imperfect, and all the better for that. This feeling is prompted by a natural beauty, that which is austere and unadorned.

The closest term we have for this response in the English language is "aesthetic arrest," as hinted at by James Joyce in his novel *A Portrait of the Artist as a Young Man*.[17] Joyce wrote,

> The instant wherein that supreme quality of beauty, the clear radiance of the esthetic image, is apprehended luminously by the mind which has been arrested by its wholeness and fascinated by its harmony is the luminous silent stasis of esthetic pleasure, a spiritual state very like to that cardiac condition which the Italian physiologist Luigi Galvani ... called the enchantment of the heart.

But even this is just talking about the physical response, and not the deeper philosophy of *wabi sabi*, which relates to the nature of life itself.

Life lessons inspired by *wabi sabi*

Wabi sabi is deeply connected to the kind of beauty that reminds us of the transient nature of life. This stems from the three Buddhist marks of existence: *mujō* (無常, impermanence), *ku* (苦, suffering), and *kū* (空, no individual self, a oneness with all things).

The life lessons *wabi sabi* can teach us, and that we will explore in this book, are rooted in the following ideas:

- The world looks very different when you learn to see and experience it from your heart.
- All things, including life itself, are impermanent, incomplete, and imperfect. Therefore, perfection is impossible,

and imperfection is the natural state of everything, including ourselves.

- There is great beauty, value, and comfort to be found in simplicity.

Still, *wabi sabi* is not a panacea. It's a reminder that stillness, simplicity, and beauty can help us fully inhabit a moment in the middle of anything, and that's a lesson for all of us.

A NOTE ABOUT LANGUAGE

Based on some of what has been written about *wabi sabi* by non-Japanese people in the past, you might have heard it used as an adjective—as in "a *wabi sabi* bowl," in the same way you might say "a wonky teacup" or a "weathered chair." In the West it has come to describe a particular natural and imperfect look. However, it's important to know that Japanese people do not use the term *wabi sabi* in this way.

At a stretch you might get away with saying something "has an air of *wabi sabi*" or "gives you a feeling of *wabi sabi*," but the term itself—at least in the original Japanese—does not describe the external look of an object. Rather, it conveys the impression you are left with after an encounter with a particular kind of beauty, which may be visual but could be experiential.

An ex-professor I talked to singled out the appreciation of moss in the garden of an old temple as a time he gets a feeling of *wabi sabi*. For a taxi-driving saxophonist I met, it is when he plays the blues. For others it was in the context of the tea ceremony. It varies from person to person, because we are all moved by different things. But the moment this feeling arises—a knowing, a connection, a reminder of the evanescent and imperfect nature of life itself—then *wabi sabi* is present.

The meaning of words often shifts when they are brought into other languages, so if you have been using *wabi sabi* as an adjective and it helps you treasure imperfection and the simple life, then it's not something to worry about. The point of this book is not to get caught up in semantics but rather to extricate life lessons inspired by this wisdom, to soak up the philosophy and be moved by it to change your viewpoint in a way that enhances your life.

Indeed, it is not to say we cannot use the concept of *wabi sabi* to inspire the way we arrange our homes to honor simplicity, nature, and beauty. We can, and we will go into this in depth in chapter 2. But if we pigeonhole *wabi sabi* simply as a desirable lifestyle or design trend, we miss the real opportunity offered by this deep and intuitive way of experiencing the world.

One of the most intriguing and simultaneously challenging things about Japanese language and culture is their layering. Nothing is ever quite as it seems. Everything depends on the context, on who is speaking to whom and what has been left unsaid. If one of the central tenets of "imperfection" is incompleteness, my job here is to paint a rich yet incomplete picture of *wabi sabi*, so you can fill in the blanks from your own perspective.

In some parts of this book, I will speak purely of *wabi sabi*. In others, I will bring in related concepts from Japan that contribute to a simpler yet richer way of life. Ultimately, I hope you will come to sense the essence of *wabi sabi* for yourself and welcome it into your own life as inspiration for a new way of beholding the world.

A gift for us all

Not long ago, I watched a pair of Japanese high school students give a presentation on *wabi sabi* in the United States. At the end, one of the Americans in the audience asked, "Do you think anyone can learn *wabi sabi*?" The girls looked at each other, brows crinkled, panicked and unsure. After much deliberation, one of them responded, "No. We feel it because we are Japanese."

❀

Wabi sabi invites us to be present to beauty with open eyes and an open heart.

I disagree. *Wabi sabi* is a deeply human response to beauty that I believe we all have the capacity to experience, if only we better attune ourselves to it.

My perspective on *wabi sabi* will always be in the context of my own worldview, which is based on a Western upbringing, heavily influenced by a twenty-year love affair with Japan. Your perspective will differ from mine, and if you have the opportunity to talk to a Japanese person about it, their perspective will be different again. But therein lies the beauty and largely the point—it is in taking inspiration from other cultures and interpreting it in the context of our own lives that we excavate the wisdom we most need.

How is *wabi sabi* relevant today?

We are living in a time of brain-hacking algorithms, pop-up propaganda, and information everywhere. From the moment we wake up to the time we stumble into bed, we are fed messages about what we should look like, wear, eat, and buy, how much we should be earning, who we should love, and how we should parent. Many of us probably spend more time thinking about other people's lives than investing in our own. Add to this the pace at which we are encouraged to function, and it's no wonder so many of us are feeling overwhelmed, insecure, untethered, and worn out.

What's more, we are surrounded by bright, artificial light, in our homes, stores, and offices, and on our phones and laptops. We are overstimulated and obsessed with productivity. It's playing havoc with our nervous systems and ability to sleep. We are paying the price of having banished the calming shadows and rich texture from our lives, in favor of speed and efficiency. Our eyes and hearts are weary.

> We give away freely that most precious of resources—our attention—and in doing so, we cheat ourselves out of the gifts that are already here.

While powerful and valuable in many ways, social media is turning us into comparison addicts and validation junkies. We interrupt precious life moments to take a picture and post it, then spend the next hour checking how much approval we have received from people we hardly even know. Any time we have a spare minute, out comes the phone and down go the eyes as we scroll our way into someone else's highly styled life, the jealousy bubbling as we make the assumption that they actually live like that. Every time we do this, we miss unknowable opportunities for connection, serendipity, and everyday adventure in our own lives, for the mind has gone somewhere the body cannot follow.

Many of us can't make a move without stressing about what others will think. We stand in line waiting for permission from somebody else, all the while worrying about things that haven't yet happened. We tell ourselves stories about our limits, downplaying where we measure up and overplaying where we fall short.

When we dare to imagine following our dreams, we are surrounded by so many manicured images of success that we start wondering whether there's any room left for us. Countless broken dreams lie scattered across the world for no reason other than someone compared themselves to someone else and thought, "I am not good enough." The upshot of this crisis of confidence is, at best, inertia.

Somewhere along the line, someone started a rumor that happiness lies in the accumulation of things, money, power, and status, all the while looking young, pretty, and skinny, or young, handsome, and strong. But when we measure our lives with other people's yardsticks, opening ourselves up to the tyranny of "should," we put ourselves under immense pressure to achieve, to do and own stuff we don't really care about. This desire for more affects our behavior, our decision making, and the way we feel about ourselves—not to mention the impact on our planet. Whatever we have or become, it's not enough, or so we are led to believe.

And here's the real irony. What we outwardly push for is often very different to what we inwardly long for. We have come to a point where we need to pause, take a look around, and decide for ourselves what really matters. *Wabi sabi* can help us do this, which makes this centuries-old teaching more relevant today than ever.

A new way

What we need right now is a new way of seeing the world and our place within it.

We need new approaches to life's challenges. We need tools

for intentional and conscious living and a framework for deciding what really matters to us, so we can move on from the constant desire for more, better, best. We need to find ways to slow down, so life does not rush right past us. We need to start noticing more beauty to lift our spirits and keep us inspired. We need to give ourselves permission to let go of judgment and the endless pursuit of perfection. And we need to start seeing one another—and ourselves—for the perfectly imperfect treasures that we are.

All this, that we so desperately need, can be found in the philosophy of *wabi sabi*. Not because it solves the surface problems, but because it can fundamentally shift the way we see life itself. *Wabi sabi* teaches us to be content with less, in a way that feels like more:

> Less stuff, more soul. Less hustle, more ease. Less chaos, more calm.
> Less mass consumption, more unique creation.
> Less complexity, more clarity. Less judgment, more forgiveness. Less bravado, more truth.
> Less resistance, more resilience. Less control, more surrender. Less head, more heart.

Letting go of what you think should be does not mean giving up on what could be.

Wabi sabi represents a precious cache of wisdom that values tranquility, harmony, beauty, and imperfection, and can strengthen our resilience in the face of modern ills.

More important, accepting imperfection doesn't mean having to lower standards or drop out of life. It means not judging yourself for being who you are: perfectly imperfect—at once uniquely you and just like the rest of us.

Put simply, *wabi sabi* gives you permission to be yourself. It encourages you to do your best but not make yourself ill in pursuit of an unattainable goal of perfection. It gently motions you to relax, slow down, and enjoy your life. And it shows you that beauty can be found in the most unlikely of places, making every day a doorway to delight.

質素簡潔

CHAPTER 2:
SIMPLIFYING +
BEAUTIFYING

Given Japan's mountainous nature, with forests, fields, and agricultural land covering some 80 percent of the country,[1] it's no surprise that the nation's urban areas are crowded. Tōkyō has a population of more than thirteen million,[2] with more than six thousand people per square kilometer.[3] As a result, the Japanese have become masters of small-space architecture and styling.

Personal space is limited and, in recent years, clutter has become as much of a challenge for the Japanese people as it has for many of us in other nations. Perhaps this is why they have become so adept at organization and storage, why Muji (literally, "no label") is a shopping district favorite, and why Marie Kondō is a household name. However, don't be fooled into thinking that most Japanese people now live in tatami-matted rooms[4] devoid of stuff. They don't. While the overall concept of minimalism has had a transformative impact for many, it can end up being another kind of perfection. It's one more opportunity to beat yourself up for not doing something right, and frankly, it's exhausting.

Perhaps you're like me. You like the philosophy of minimalism and have entertained dreams of a perfectly tidy home, but found that disciplined minimalism doesn't really work for you because you have children/pets/a hectic lifestyle/a weird fetish for antique teapots/more books than your local library or some other reason that makes you run from perfectly organized sock drawers. Or perhaps you rent and are limited in terms of how you are allowed to alter your living space. Or maybe you are on a tight budget and think that a welcoming home is for people with more disposable income. Or maybe you are just busy, and it feels like such an effort to go through everything. If any of this sounds familiar, the alternative "soulful simplicity" might just be for you.

A *wabi sabi* lens can inspire us to embrace soulful simplicity and treasure what we already have.

"Soulful simplicity" is my name for decluttering and styling your home with love, without making it clinically minimal or trying too hard. It's a way of organizing and personalizing your space, which makes your home welcoming and beautiful while still feeling lived in.

There is a lovely phrase in Japanese, *igokochi ga yoi* (居心地が良い). The kanji[5] literally mean "being here–heart–place–good," and it is used to describe a feeling of comfort, of feeling at home. I like to think of it as a place for a happy heart. That's what we want to create with soulful simplicity.

Your home, your space

The spaces in which we live influence *the way* in which we live and how we feel as we go about our daily lives. If we want to live differently, changing our environment, and the details of our living spaces, can play a major role in making a shift. Our homes can be sanctuaries; gathering places; repositories of love and laughter, solitude and rest. They can be grounding, comforting, inspiring, and relaxing. Our homes are where our stories are written, and they have the potential to enhance our experience of the everyday.

The beauty of soulful simplicity is that it can help us make any dwelling—regardless of size or budget—a lovely place to be. This comes as a relief to those of us who swoon over design magazines and lose hours on Pinterest and Instagram but have the niggling feeling that our homes will never quite look like that. *Wabi sabi* reminds us that they are not supposed to look like that. Homes are for living in, and living is not a perfectly tidy affair. The good news is that the chaos of real life, edited a little, can reveal a lot. Most of us already have the makings of a welcoming space. With just a little time and attention, your home can become a sanctuary reflecting what really matters to you.

A *wabi sabi*–inspired home: lived in, loved, and never quite finished.

Taking inspiration from the traditional tearoom—the embodiment of *wabi sabi*—we can envision a clean, simple, uncluttered space. It's about deciding what to retain and what to release, what to show and what to store, what to tinker with and what to treasure.

You don't need to wait for the perfect time—when you have the money to redecorate, when your children have left home, or when you finally have time to sort every drawer and closet. You can begin today, right where you are. This is not a set of rules; it's a set of ideas and questions for you to consider in order to do it your way.

The emotional connection

The truth is that many of us have houses filled with clutter, even though we don't like it. We buy stuff when we don't need it. We tell ourselves we really should get everything in order and then we switch on the TV instead. During the years in my work with people trying to make major life changes, decluttering has always

Soulful simplicity makes for contented sufficiency.

been a significant part of their journey. As they begin to release more and more stuff, they begin to notice the releasing of negative thought patterns, feelings of insufficiency, allegiances to busyness, attachments to past versions of themselves, and desires for a life that is not connected to who they are or what they really value. This is where *wabi sabi* really comes in.

When you realize you are perfectly imperfect just as you are, you have less need for "stuff" to boost your self-image. Ultimately, soulful simplicity in your home is about you and the experience you want to create for yourself, your family, and your friends. This is about tuning in to what you love and making space for authentic inspiration. It's about what pulls you in. It's about quality, depth, and choice. And it's about putting your judgment to one side and focusing on what you can do with what you already have.

A *wabi sabi*–inspired home is a restful space that welcomes guests and nourishes family life. It's a place for treasured things that carry love and evoke memories, not just new things bought on impulse. There is no right or wrong. It's unpretentious styling, done in a perfectly imperfect way.

Later in this chapter I will introduce some tips for decluttering and soulfully simplifying your space in a *wabi sabi*–inspired way. But first let's take a look at the notion of Japanese beauty that lies beneath it all.

Making beauty

If you were to put your nose against the glass and peer through the window of the old shed studio, you might see Makiko Hastings at her potter's wheel, sitting on a wooden chair flecked with slip and marked with the ghostly fingerprints of an artisan at work. You'd notice her shoulders rise and fall in gentle rhythm as she ushers the clay into shape. On the shelves behind her, you'd see rows of drying pieces, each handcrafted with love and her innate sense of beauty.

I first came to know Makiko's work seven years ago when I bought a set of the bird-shaped chopstick rests she made to raise funds for the victims of the Great East Japan Earthquake back in 2011. In all, she made more than a thousand ceramic birds to support the residents of the town of Minamisanriku, which was 70 percent destroyed by the tsunami that followed the earthquake. Makiko has had her own share of challenges over the years, but she has come out the other side with a deep appreciation for her family and for her creativity.

These days, Makiko crafts each of her pieces with individual care, for her online shop[6] and trade customers. Asked about her aesthetic choices, she explains how simplicity in one area allows for detail in another. One example is a set of dinner plates she was recently commissioned to make for the head chef of a Yorkshire restaurant. Unusually flat, they have an exquisite cobalt glaze that varies slightly from plate to plate, giving each diner a unique visual experience of their food.

Beyond her consideration of the form, decoration, and color, Makiko sees her plates as a receptacle not just for food but also for memories. Crucially, she believes that the customer completes the beauty of each piece by using and treasuring it. And therein lies a crucial observation: Japanese beauty is discovered in the experiencing, not just the seeing.

Deconstructing Japanese beauty

There is no single agreed-on set of terms to define Japanese beauty, so I have curated the most popular ideas with the aim of making it easily translatable into your life. On the surface of Japanese beauty there is taste (the visual); beneath it is flavor (the experience).

Consider for a moment some of the things we might associate with beauty in Japan: the striking elegance of a *maiko* (apprentice geisha)[7] in her sumptuous chartreuse silk kimono, paired with an intricately embroidered scarlet obi;[8] the chic look of a smart Tōkyōite; the artfulness of a single camellia in an ash-glazed *Hagi-yaki*[9] vase or the simplicity of a traditional tatami mat room. How are all these views of Japan—so different in style, color, texture, pattern, and complexity—part of the same aesthetic construct? It all comes down to taste.

The beauty on the surface

If we were to mark out the key types of Japanese taste on a spectrum it would look something like this:

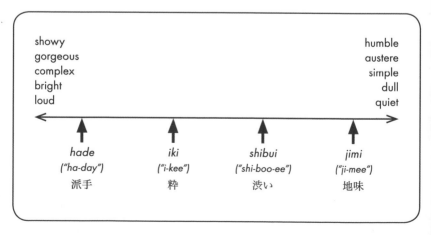

showy	humble
gorgeous	austere
complex	simple
bright	dull
loud	quiet

hade ("ha-day") 派手 | *iki* ("i-kee") 粋 | *shibui* ("shi-boo-ee") 渋い | *jimi* ("ji-mee") 地味

Hade (派手)   Showy, gaudy, liberal. A bright kimono, bejeweled nails, high-color manga characters. The colors can be anything from primaries to neons.

Iki (粋)   Chic, stylish, worldly, and sophisticated. The appearance of being effortlessly cool (although it may have taken some effort); think sharp suits and sophisticated officewear, confident use of color.

Shibui (渋い)   Sometimes translated as austere, subdued, subtle, or restrained, although "to the Japanese the word is more complex, suggesting quietness, depth, simplicity and purity."[10] In recent times, *shibui* has come to mean something closer to quietly cool, well-designed, understated style. In terms of colors, it suggests dark, rich, and deep, often with some neutrals and a hint of a dusty accent color, like the palette of a hydrangea.[11]

Jimi (地味)   Literally means "earth taste"—sober, conservative, unobtrusive. Neutral, beige, or dull gray tones. If patterned, a low-contrast all-over plain design.

There is a place for elegance in each of these tastes, but they look very different on the surface. They can also be used to describe attitudes.

Where does *wabi sabi* fit in?

For some time now the term *wabi sabi* has been used in the West as an adjective to describe a particular taste. It has come to represent a natural, rustic look, which honors imperfection, organic materials, textures, and character. In terms of colors, think subtle

shades of nature—earth tones, greens, blues, neutrals, grays, rusts.
I love objects with characteristics like these. I am drawn to them
and I decorate my home with them. But they are not *wabi sabi* in
the deep sense that we have been discussing.

My guess is that this shift in meaning happened some time
ago, when some daring foreigners, intrigued by *wabi sabi*, sought
to get to the heart of the matter. I imagine the kindly Japanese
people they asked about it perhaps couldn't find the right words,
so instead they pointed to things like a simple bowl, a tea-
ceremony room, or a withered leaf—things they associate with
the experience of *wabi sabi* but that are not intrinsically so. As a
result, we have come to a curious place where many of us non-
Japanese are familiar with *wabi sabi* as a name for a particular look
that celebrates imperfection and the mark of time, rather than
appreciating its powerful depths.

To avoid confusion, and for want of a single Japanese word, I
will use the term "*wabisabi*esque" to describe this particular kind
of visual taste (on the surface), in contrast to the philosophical
wabi sabi as an experience of the essence of beauty (in the depths).

Here are some of the terms most commonly used to describe
the *wabisabi*esque look:

- Asymmetrical
- Atmospheric
- Flawed beauty
- Humble
- Imperfect
- Irregular
- Marked by the passage of time
- Modest
- Natural

- Nostalgic
- Organic
- Raw
- Restrained
- Rough
- Rustic
- Serene
- Simple
- Soulful
- Subtle
- Textured
- Understated

If we were then to add this *wabisabi*esque to the taste spectrum, I think it would sit somewhere between *shibui* and *jimi* (although exactly where it sits is, of course, a matter of taste):

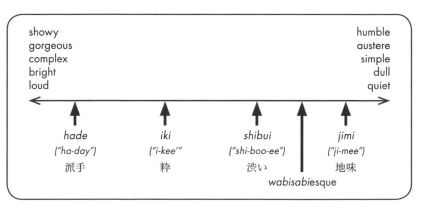

showy	humble
gorgeous	austere
complex	simple
bright	dull
loud	quiet

hade
("ha-day")
派手

iki
("i-kee'")
粋

shibui
("shi-boo-ee")
渋い

jimi
("ji-mee")
地味

*wabisabi*esque

What is your natural style?

Take a moment to consider where your natural taste lies on this spectrum. To help you identify this, take a look around your own home and think about the kind of spaces that inspire you. Remember, visual interest can come from texture, shape, scale, and shadow, not just from color.

- **If your taste is *hade* or *iki*,** *wabisabi*esque style can add a little calm and serenity, and help you reconnect with nature.
- **If your taste is *shibui*,** *wabisabi*esque style is likely a natural fit for you, if not already on your radar, and can bring a little more character and story.
- **If your taste is *jimi*,** *wabisabi*esque style can add a little warmth and richness.

The beauty beneath

The Japanese appreciation of beauty does not stop at the external. Rather, there are particular words to describe the emotional quality of beauty beneath the surface, connected to our experience of that beauty. There is a host of different words to represent different aspects of this, some of which cross over in meaning with others. To keep it simple I would like to share just the most important ones here.[12]

Mono no aware (物の哀れ)

The term *mono no aware* is a refined sensitivity and emotional response to time-limited beauty, and has been variously translated as "the pathos of things," "the bittersweet poignancy of things," and even "the aah-ness of things." It is the beauty in perishability. At first glance, the description may seem similar to ideas about *wabi sabi*, but there is one distinct difference: *mono no aware* focuses on the beauty (and the impending vanishing of that beauty), whereas *wabi sabi* draws our attention to what that beauty reminds us about life. When Japanese people use metaphors to describe each term, they will often reference the fleeting beauty of the delicate blooming pink cherry blossom just before it falls when alluding to *mono no aware*, but for *wabi sabi* they would be more likely to speak of a fallen autumn leaf.

Yūgen (幽玄)

The term *yūgen* refers to the depth of the world as seen with our imagination. It has been likened to the beauty of grace, of mystery, and of realizing we are a small part of something so much greater than ourselves. *Yūgen* is considered one of the most important principles of traditional Japanese Nōh drama. It emerged from the highly refined culture of the Heian-era nobility[13] and has evolved over time to represent a profound sense of wonder instilled by the poetic nature of beauty.

Wabi (侘)

As we saw in chapter 1, *wabi* is the feeling generated by recognizing the beauty found in simplicity. It is a sense of quiet contentment found away from the trappings of a materialistic world. The spirit of *wabi* is deeply connected to the idea of accepting that our true needs are quite simple, and of being humble and grateful for the beauty that already exists right where we are.

Sabi (寂)

Again, as we saw in chapter 1, *sabi* communicates a deep and tranquil beauty that emerges with the passage of time. Visually, we recognize this as the patina of age, weathering, tarnishing, and signs of antiquity and, as such, it can be used to describe the appearance of a thing. But it also goes deeper than that. It is a particular beauty that respects, reflects, and reminds us of the natural cycle of life, prompting a host of emotional responses ranging from wistfulness and melancholy to pensiveness and longing.

These emotional elements of beauty are of great importance to the Japanese aesthetic sense. To appreciate them, we have to pause, pay attention, be open, and tune in.

Writing about Japanese beauty in *House Beautiful* in 1958, then editor Elizabeth Gordon, who was in the process of a five-year-long research project preparing for two record-breaking issues on Japan, said:

> First, you won't learn to recognize beauty if you are tied to the familiar or the time-honored way of doing something. You have to look at everything through pure eyes, which means forgetting all associations of price, age, social context, prestige, etc. Wipe away all judgments made by others and respond to the object as you do to those things in nature such as trees, sunsets, clouds and mountains. Second, you won't learn to see beauty if you look at objects isolated from each other. Especially in objects inescapably tied to each other. Things grow or shrink in beauty depending on what environment they are seen against.[14]

Inspired by Japan, one of America's leading tastemakers at the time hereby gave her readers blanket permission to stop judging the things they put in their home by their perceived value in relation to what others thought and rather to embrace what instinctively drew them in.

The beauty inside

Japanese beauty cannot be described, in one word, with logic. It has to be seen with the eye and the heart, participated in, experienced. The most important lesson *wabi sabi* teaches us for inviting more beauty into our lives and living spaces is this:

Beauty is in the heart of the beholder.

But if beauty is in the *heart* of the beholder, what does this mean in practice for us, in terms of discovering a new way of seeing?

It means seeking out beauty with all our senses. It means pulling ourselves back from the constant pursuit of more, so we can notice what's already in our field of vision. It means slowing down enough to look and paying attention to what lies beneath the surface. It means surrounding ourselves with things and people and ideas we love and cherish. And it means reflecting, every now and then, on the fact that life is a cycle, not a forever, and that it's short and precious.

千畳敷に寝ても畳一枚
Senjyōjiki ni nete mo tatami ichi mai.
Even in a room of a thousand tatami mats, you only sleep on one.
—*Japanese proverb*

It also means opening our hearts to possibility and wonder. And it means looking for the gifts of a simpler life.

Making your home your own

Spread around me on the floor is a multitude of interior magazines and books I have collected from Japan over the years. I am trying to pinpoint exactly what it is that has long drawn me to Japanese design and style. As my eyes flit across the covers and my hands flip through the pages, I am transported back to the early 2000s, when I was living and working in Tōkyō. I had a hectic job in the world of sports, but in my spare moments—at lunchtimes and on weekends—I would spend hours in cozy cafés, reading about architecture, interior design, ceramics, textiles, and styling. Rare days off were spent visiting exhibitions and seeking out independent shops in Jiyūgaoka, Daikanyama, and Kagurazaka, delighting not only in the beautifully crafted products on offer but also in the way they were packaged and wrapped.

When considering what to do after my contract had ended, I mulled over the prospect of training as an "interior coordinator," helping people style their homes. There was a huge boom in *zakka* shops. The rather dull translation of *zakka* as "miscellaneous items" belies the delight found in *zakka* treasures—things that express your taste and personality and add layers of story to your home. Many of the products in *zakka* shops were compact, reflecting both the Japanese love of attention to detail and the practical reality of people living in small spaces. Around this time, I developed a slight obsession with Japanese stationery, a love that continues to this day. I also discovered the Japanese genius for home organization and creative storage.

My tiny apartment in Ushigome-Yanagichō was tucked away in a quiet patch of residential houses, far from the nearest highrise, which made the area feel more like a village than the middle of a thriving metropolis. The front door opened into a *genkan* (entranceway) where shoes would be removed before stepping up into the apartment. With the exception of a small bathroom, my place was a one-room studio. Outside the kitchen window was a small disused piece of land where mint grew like wildfire. To this day, I think of the apartment every time I smell that cool, refreshing scent.

I furnished it slowly and carefully, on a budget and within the constraints that come with such a modest space. Each item was treasured and had a memory attached. The *washi* paper I used as a wall hanging had been sourced from my favorite paper shop one early spring afternoon, just as the plum blossom was falling. The linen tablemats, hand-carved chopsticks, and well-loved crockery had been precious gifts from friends. I used them even when it was just me for dinner, which was most days.

Books about flowers, pottery, and slow living were stacked in small piles with a teapot or a vase atop, used as decorations in place of expensive *objets*.

These days, we have so much choice and access to so many cheap things, we usually shop, consume, and grow our credit-card bills in a hurry. Our lives and our closets are rapidly becoming overstuffed. In recent years, as my family has grown to include two young daughters with a penchant for pink plastic and baby dolls, I have found myself returning to Japanese inspiration for ideas on bringing a sense of serenity to our home without breaking the bank.

Before we can beautify, we need to simplify and make the most of the space that we have.

Themes to inspire you

To come back to the commonalities between the Japanese interior design books and magazines that lay scattered at my feet, I noticed several threads: simple clear spaces, texture in furnishings, carefully chosen items displayed in a way that is gentle on the eye, small things in a small place (no oversize furniture, for example), more things put away than on display, nature indoors (from a tiny courtyard garden to flowers and found objects displayed inside),

and a sense of the seasons, shadows and light, lots of neutrals, flexibility in the way the space is used, and an underlying sense of calm.

There was also often a detail that invited a sense of wonder. A
single bloom in a tiny vase. A partly hidden view, suggesting but
not telling. This made me think about how we could benefit from
not putting all our treasures on display, not cramming every spare
inch with stuff, not telling our whole life story on first meeting
or rushing to fill all the pauses in a conversation.

I have gathered these threads into five themes for you to
explore in your own life. They are: simplicity, space, flexibility,
nature, and details.[15]

Simplicity

One Japanese lifestyle brand I have admired for years is Fog Linen
Work,[16] founded by designer and entrepreneur Yumiko Sekine
more than two decades ago. Her store, tucked away on a small street
in the trendy Shimo-Kitazawa district of Tōkyō, is a serene oasis
in the bustling capital. Exposed concrete walls are a textured yet
neutral backdrop for wide-open shelves, which hold linen napkins
in wire baskets, small stacks of wooden plates, and open trays with
tiny buttons. Linen clothing and bags in subtle colors are spread out
on a long rail. My favorite items are the heavy-duty aprons, which
make you want to go straight home and cook something. There
is a sense of space, and of time stopping inside the store.

Sekine-*san* has had years of exposure to the West, having
imported lifestyle goods from the United States before she set up
Fog, and now working primarily with Lithuanian suppliers to
manufacture the linen goods she herself designs. This makes her
style choices even more accessible, as they seem just as at home
in a San Francisco apartment or a London town house as in a
Japanese abode.

When asked to share a few words about her particular style she told me:

> It's simple, minimal, organized. My European distributor tells me there is something distinctly Japanese about the way I display our products. I like calm neutrals, and I sometimes use accent colors for our clothes, depending on the season. My aim is to make quiet products that can ease themselves into people's lives and homes, bringing a subtle sense of calm. I like to live with natural materials, such as linen, cotton, wood, and some metal. No plastic. This suits my personality and my love of simple things.

Every time I go to Sekine-*san*'s store it inspires me to make my own shelves more open, to pare back and display only things I really love. When we stop using shelves just for storage and instead see them as holders of treasures, the difference is remarkable. Instead of a room closing in on you, it seems to open up.

On my return from Tōkyō this time, I hung my linen apron on a hook where I could see it, made a simple display of cookbooks paired with vintage bottles and old photos on the windowsill, shook out a favorite tablecloth, and popped some wildflowers in a vase to go in the center of the table. It took a couple of minutes and cost me nothing. Instantly, I wanted to be in the kitchen, making something delicious for my little family.

Top tips for decluttering

It is well documented that decluttering our spaces can help declutter our minds, not to mention save us time and money. Try it in your own home with these simple tips:

1. First, taking inspiration from the household-organization guru Marie Kondō,[17] make a list of the main categories of "stuff" in your home, such as books or toys. Then pick a category and gather like things together from all around the house. Select only what you need or truly love and then get rid of the rest (sell, recycle, donate). This can be fairly daunting if you have stuff spread all over your house, but in the end it means you are making decisions based on all the facts. When you realize you have five sun hats but only go somewhere hot once a year, it suddenly becomes easier to let go of excess stuff. When putting the remaining items away, try to keep like things together, so you can easily retrieve them.

2. Consider what you can replace or eliminate with technology—for example, using music apps instead of buying physical recordings, printing and framing a few special photos and storing the rest digitally, or perhaps using e-readers and the local library for all but your favorite books.

3. Consider what you can store in your memory instead of in your closets. For example, if a distant relative passed away and you received a box full of items connected with them, choose one thing to keep as a reminder and then release the rest.

4. Gather up your paper mountain and sort it into three piles: (a) To Action; (b) To File; and (c) To Toss. With pile (a) To Action, set aside an afternoon where you action every single item. No excuses. With pile (b) To File, where possible scan and digitally store and back up your documents, and then shred the originals, keeping only what is required by law, such as home-ownership documents. With pile (c) To Toss, shred anything private and recycle the rest. Then choose one place where you will put all pending paper from now on and make a weekly appointment with yourself to action, file, or toss.

5. One dropped piece of clothing, unfiled letter, or dumped toy is a magnet for others. Bring in a simple system for easy tidiness.
6. Involve those you live with. Make it a game.
7. Don't forget to declutter your handbag or wallet. It's a space you probably view more times in a day than most of the rooms in your house.

Space

Although the average Japanese person does not live in an architect-designed home, there are valuable lessons to be learned from the principles of Japanese architecture to inspire our own spaces. To discover more about these, I sought out Dr. Teruaki Matsuzaki, one of Japan's foremost architectural historians, who outlined the main characteristics of Japanese architecture as follows:

- *Ma* (間, space)[18]
- Nature and the connection between inside and outside
- A sense of beauty
- An understanding of light and shadow
- The careful selection of materials (quality, source, texture, smell)
- The concept of "less is more"

Reiterating Makiko's feelings about her pottery clients playing a role in the beauty of her products, Matsuzaki-*sensei* said that the key to aesthetic genius is leaving something unfinished to draw the viewer in. Beautiful writing leaves something unsaid, so the reader can finish it in their imagination. Beautiful art leaves something unexplained, so the viewer participates with their curiosity. It's the same with architecture and interiors. Perfection and completeness are not the ideal, even if architecture appears "perfect" in design magazines. Matsuzaki-*sensei* said, "Spaces are ultimately created to be lived in and used, and if they don't do that well, they are not considered successful."

What can we take from this for our own homes? We can create space. We can bring nature in. We can decide what we consider to be beautiful and integrate that. We can be aware not just of light but also of shadow. We can choose the materials we use carefully, and we can make choices that leave us living with what we really love.

MAKING SPACE, ONE ROOM AT A TIME

The satisfaction of early results breeds enthusiasm, so I'm a big believer in first tackling what you most often see. First, declutter main items (books, clothes, toys, files, etc.), using the tips in this chapter. Then try some of these ideas in one room at a time, in your home or workspace:

1. Clear everything from the floor.
2. Clear everything from the surfaces.
3. Clear everything from the walls.
4. Now add things back in slowly, asking yourself the following questions:
   - How do I want to feel when I am in this room? What color palette will help me feel that way? (Consider the spectrum of taste shared in this chapter, and how *wabisabi*esque style and colors could bring a sense of calm, warmth, and character to the room.)
   - What do I like about this emptier space? Which aspects of it would I like to keep clear? (If you feel like repainting, now would be a good time.)

- What could I do differently on the walls? What would be special? What has meaning or memory? (Examples of interesting things to frame include maps, postcards, inspiring words, children's art, your art, posters, a tea towel or scarf, a sheet of beautiful wrapping paper, dried flowers.)
- How can I arrange the furniture to make the best use of the space? Is this the right furniture for the room? (Now might be a good time to sell something that doesn't work for you, and visit a flea market, antiques shop, or independent furniture maker for ideas for a replacement, or try upcycling something yourself.)
- What particular items do I already own that can bring beauty into this room? What adds a sense of story? What can I repurpose? Add these back in slowly, in small groups for interest.
- How can I bring nature into this room and introduce more natural materials? How can I reflect the season?
- How can I bring in texture (with fabric, paper, rough finishes, for example) on the walls, the furniture, the floor, the ceiling?
- If you enjoy books, how can you include them as display items? (On shelves, stacked to make a side table, three high with something on top to make a small arrangement, for example.)

5. Now look at all the other objects you removed from the room, which you have chosen not to put back. Use the tips in this chapter to declutter and sort them.

6. Make a note in your diary to swap things around and refresh this room once every season, or monthly if you prefer.

7. When you're ready, enjoy a cup of tea or coffee in your beautiful space, then move on to the next room!

Flexibility

For those people who live in more traditional Japanese dwellings, usually in the suburbs or rural areas, their homes tend to be made primarily of wood. Walls are thin and often flexible to allow for best use of space. Tatami-matted rooms are often multipurpose, transitioning from a relaxation space, to a meditation space, to an eating space, to a sleeping space. You can move doors and tables, lay the futon out or put it away, host people or retreat from them.

To find out more about this idea of flexibility, I spent some time in the home of my friend Daisuke Sanada, CEO of Suwa Architects and Designers. The son of a carpenter himself, Sanada-*san* built his home with a little help from several carpenter friends, in a small town on the outskirts of Tōkyō. He lives with his wife, Sayaka, who is an interior designer, and their family in a compact, well-thought-out, beautiful space.

Sanada-*san*, who is descended from a famous samurai warrior, has a strong sense of tradition and vast knowledge of his country's heritage. He brings this to his work, along with a contemporary eye and a love of cozy spaces, which help to strengthen the bonds of the people living in them.

His own home is over two stories, the front part double height with a carefully handcrafted pitched cedar roof and a huge triangular window at one end, which makes the trees outside feel like they are part of the house. This open area houses the living, dining, and cooking spaces, with a raised section of tatami alongside a wood-fired stove creating the perfect place for his dog to curl up, for doing some morning yoga, or for catching a nap on a winter's afternoon. A simple wooden sideboard plays host to a relaxed display of crumbling Yayoi-period pots dug up in his friend's rice field. In the region of two thousand years old, they have been repurposed as simple vases and brought into the

Sanada family's daily life to enjoy rather than being stored away like museum pieces.

At the back of the ground floor are a bathroom, bedroom, and storage room, with a ladder leading up to the chill-out area and another sleeping space on the mezzanine above. This upper section is divided up using flexible furniture, such as moveable bookcases and fabric curtains hung from the ceiling, to allow for privacy or company, depending on the day. The result is a welcoming home that supports the lifestyle Sanada-*san* and his family want. It is stylish, yet practical, and soulfully simple.

Sanada-*san* and I spent many hours talking about the value of contrast and relationship in Japanese life: how beauty is found in the existence of tension; light and shadow; sound and silence; simplicity and detail; sublime and ordinary; presence and absence; freedom and restraint; *wabi* and *sabi*. We talked about how beauty often arises in the middle of things—a conversation, a lifetime, a walk in the woods. And how everything is connected—everything within a space, the inside and the outside, our surroundings and our minds, in our relationships with each other and ourselves in the web of nature.

Those of us who do not live in Japanese-style homes can still be inspired by these ideas. We can divide up our spaces with the placement of our furniture, rugs, and shelving, and move things around regularly, depending on how we want to use the space, acknowledging that it is never "finished" and we aren't aiming for perfection. We can repaint walls, swap out displays, bring in some seasonal flowers and plants, and refresh whenever the mood arises. We can pay attention to the visual contrasts and the relationships between what we see and how we feel. A window is not just a window—it is a frame for all that lies beyond it. A shelf on one side of the room may be a balance for something on the other. Notice how individual things in a room affect others and how things work together, with the space, the flow, how you live, and how it makes you feel.

Remember: utility, simplicity, beauty, story.

HOW TO INSPIRE SOULFUL SHOPPING

How can you look at the spiraling excess and waste, and the poisonous culture of comparison, and decide to do things differently? How can you be quietly radical like Sen no Rikyū (see page 13)? How can you be an advocate for something that feels more real?

The most soulful shopping of all is that which costs nothing and only inflates what you own with natural beauty. Try spending time in nature, collecting gifts from the forest, or creating with your hands instead of buying.

When you are considering buying something new, ask yourself these questions:

- Do I really need it? Do I already own something that can do the job? Am I actually going to use it?
- Do I love it? Will I still want it twenty-four hours from now? A year from now? There is a beauty in longing. Can I wait a while for it, to make sure I really want it?
- Does it serve the season of life I am in right now (or in buying it, am I trying to hold on to the past or pressuring myself into a particular version of my life in the future)?
- Does it work with the other things I own?
- Will it help me use my space more flexibly?
- Is this something I could get for free by borrowing or trading?

- What am I willing to get rid of to make space for this?
- What will I have to sacrifice to pay for this? Is it worth it?
- Is it made of natural materials? If not, is there a version that is?
- Is it worth paying a little more to get a version that will last?

Nature

Nature is an essential element of a *wabi sabi*–inspired home as it connects to the deepest part of the whole *wabi sabi* philosophy, reminding us of the transient nature of life. We will explore nature and the seasons in detail in chapter 3. For now, consider how you can bring more natural materials into your home. For example, wood with a rough grain, bamboo, clay, stone, dull metals, handmade paper, or textures woven from natural fibers. One of my favorite treasures is the old wooden rice bucket we use for storing firewood. Be creative with your ideas. Upcycle. Repurpose. Spend time at flea markets and in vintage and antiques shops. Age often adds depth and beauty to natural materials, so don't assume you have to buy new.

Spontaneity is to be encouraged. I often mix up potted herbs and bottles of oil in the metal containers hanging in my kitchen. I might use *washi* tape (low-tack masking tape made from Japanese paper) to stick some fallen nature treasures onto the wall or put up a makeshift collage of photos alongside my children's bark rubbings and leaf prints.

Cut flowers can brighten up a space. Try leaving them a little longer than their peak and notice the beauty in their fading. It can also be refreshing to embrace a little wildness, using wildflowers and found objects. Even pretty weeds. Go outside and take a look at what nature is offering you in this particular season. What gifts from the forest, or wood, or hedgerow, or beach could you bring back into your home? Fallen leaves, berries, conkers, acorns, seed pods, shells, driftwood, and feathers all carry the spirit of nature and of *wabi sabi*.

Try incorporating some of these natural items into grouped displays in corners of your home, perhaps paired with a favorite book and some old glasses or your vintage typewriter and a stack of old ribbon. A sprig of winter berries in a small jug. A handful of snowdrops from your own garden. A string of fairy lights on a fallen branch.

Details

Attention to detail is something you notice everywhere in Japan. In cafés, in shops, in homes, in temples and shrines, even in public spaces, someone has taken care to add a small detail. These details add to the interest of a space and can really make it yours.

We have a double-height window on our staircase, which used to have long, heavy curtains. They were there when we moved in, and I was loath to remove them because they looked like they had cost the previous owners a lot of money and to take them down would be a waste. But I went up and down those stairs several times a day, and every time I passed the curtains I felt a little bit resentful. In the end, I realized I was being ridiculous. It was our house now and we could use it however we wanted. So I took the curtains down.

Instantly, the hallway was flooded with natural light. In time, I would discover that at other times of the day, the windows would throw interesting shadows onto the landing. Now that we could see the deep, wide windowsill, I unwrapped an old, mottled ceramic sake bottle, gifted from a friend when I left Japan, and repurposed it as a vase with a single flower from the garden. Next to it I set out pebbles from the beach, treasure hunted by small hands on a windy day, and I finished it off with a simple postcard that said "There is a lot of beauty in ordinary things."

My little arrangement sits on the right-hand side of the windowsill, with empty space on the left. Every now and then, I'll swap out the flower and the postcard, pile up the stones or move them around. It is my kind of beautiful and offers a moment of stillness every time I go up or down the stairs.

Where could you create pockets of serenity and beauty around your home?

TEN PRINCIPLES FOR A *WABI SABI*–INSPIRED HOME

Below is a summary of my ten key principles for a *wabi sabi*–inspired home. While *wabisabi*esque objects have a role to play, they are not the full picture. The philosophy of *wabi sabi* is the guide here. It's perfectly fine for your home to be a work in progress. Real life is not like design magazines. A home is to be lived in, so there's no need to wait until everything is finished before you invite your friends over to enjoy time together.

1. Make the most of your entranceway, which is called a *genkan* in Japan. Tidy out-of-season coats away. Put out some flowers. Invite visitors to leave their shoes at the door, Japan-style (and try to encourage anyone who lives with you to make it a habit). Stack shoes on shelves or in a shoebox, or perhaps under the stairs. You might want to offer guests house slippers if the floor is cold. This keeps your home cleaner and gives an immediate sense of comfort and familiarity.

2. Decluttering saves you time and money and makes space to appreciate the things you really love. However, stark minimalism is another kind of perfection. Go for soulful simplicity instead. Think clean, uncluttered, and welcoming.

3. Experiment with natural matte materials like wood, clay, and stone in your home, and natural fabrics for bed linen, clothing, and kitchenware. See how these bring a sense of character and calm. The eye and the imagination love imperfection, asymmetry, and nonuniform surfaces.

4. Consider how you can bring actual nature into your space, with flowers, branches, seed pods, feathers, leaves, shells, pebbles, handmade wreaths, woven baskets, and so on. Discover the joy of finding and styling these yourself, creating visual poetry with the gifts of the land and sea.

5. Keep both light and shadow in mind, noting how the contrast changes your space at different times of the day. Embrace low light and darkness when it suits the season and your mood.

6. Consider all five senses in your space. This depends on where you live and the kind of space you have, but it can include anything from opening a window for the breeze to using textured fabrics on your furniture, from diffusing essential oils to playing calming music. You can even consider the sense of taste, such as using fruits and vegetables within your simple displays or adding details to make your breakfast table feel extra special.

7. Curate things you really treasure to decorate your space and nurture it with story and memory. Think about contrasts: past and present, grounding and inspiring, ordinary and special. Where possible, be creative with what you have, or repurpose items that have had a previous life.

8. Think about the importance of relationship and visual harmony. How do things look and feel in relation to other things in the room and the space itself? What is framed by your windows and internal doorways? What is on full view and what is partly hidden, hinting at something else beyond? What different textures are bringing character and warmth to the space?

9. Create tiny corners of beauty in unexpected places. A small vase on a windowsill. A handwritten note in the bathroom. A framed photograph under the stairs.

10. Notice how you need to use the space differently depending on the season of the year and the season of your life.

Sharing your space

Writing in the nineteenth century, Lafcadio Hearn[19] famously said about Japan: "The commonest incidents of everyday life are transfigured by a courtesy at once so artless and faultless that it appears to spring directly from the heart, without any teaching."[20] This attention to the moment and the recipient's needs is at the heart of *omotenashi*, Japanese hospitality.

If you have ever spent time at a Japanese *ryokan* (traditional inn), you will know that the sense of deep relaxation comes not just from the healing waters of the cedar bath, or the cozy warmth of your futon, but from the bowing and quiet attentiveness, and the delicate care wrapped in the phrase *goyukkuri dōzo* ("Please, take your time").

Ichi-go ichi-e (一期一会) is a well-loved phrase that often appears on hanging calligraphy scrolls in the alcoves of tea-ceremony rooms. It means "this meeting, this time only" and is used to remind people to treasure this particular experience as it will never be repeated. If someone hosts you at their home in Japan, however casual the event, you will likely feel incredibly well looked after. This warmhearted and sincere hospitality is not just displayed in the food and drink you are offered but in the warmth of the welcome, the attention to detail, and the presence of the host. Your host might say, "*Dōzo, omeshi agari kudasai*" (a polite way to say "Please begin"), and you might respond with a bow and the word "*Itadakimasu*," (meaning "I humbly receive this with deep appreciation"). This ritual is a lovely way to begin a shared meal.

Wabi sabi–inspired hospitality is not about having a perfectly tidy house, all designer furniture, or perfectly well-behaved children. It's about sharing your home in a relaxed, thoughtful way and being sensitive to your guests. Having said that, we must not forget that the embodiment of *wabi sabi* is the teahouse, which is often modest, unassuming, spotlessly clean and bare other than for what has been prepared for the guests. This reminds us to make our spaces clean, uncluttered, and welcoming, as far as is possible within the context of our daily lives.

Think of the kind of words used to describe the visual *wabisabi*esque—natural, humble, understated. These are the opposite of slaving over a hot stove all night to deliver the perfect six-course gourmet dinner to impress your friends, panicking when you burn the main dish and obsessing about the fact that you forgot to make the dressing, while missing out on the real conversation.

Pay attention to small details to make your guests feel at home—their favorite drink, fresh flowers on the table, your treasured heirloom tablecloth, something nourishing to eat, cozy slippers, a blanket for stargazing on a chilly night. What really matters is paying attention, lending your ears, and sharing the moment.

WABI SABI–INSPIRED WISDOM FOR SIMPLIFYING + BEAUTIFYING

- *Beauty is in the heart of the beholder.*
- *When you realize you are perfectly imperfect already, you have less need for things to boost your self-image.*
- *Soulful simplicity is a source of delight.*

TRY IT: EXPERIMENTING WITH SOULFUL SIMPLICITY

In a notebook, jot down some thoughts about the following:

❀ How does your physical space make you feel? What is your favorite thing about it? What would you like to change?

❀ What kind of objects do you own more of than you need?

❀ What accumulation habits do you have? What life habits might these be reflecting?

❀ What kind of items do you own that you treasure and could use more in your daily life?

✳ What particular aspects of Japanese beauty and soulful simplicity inspire you? How could you bring these ideas into your own space?

✳ If you could let go of one thing in your life (material or otherwise), what would it be? What difference might that make? How could a deeper awareness of beauty and soulful simplicity support you in letting that go?

✳ What else in your life would you like to simplify?

✳ What is it that you really need?

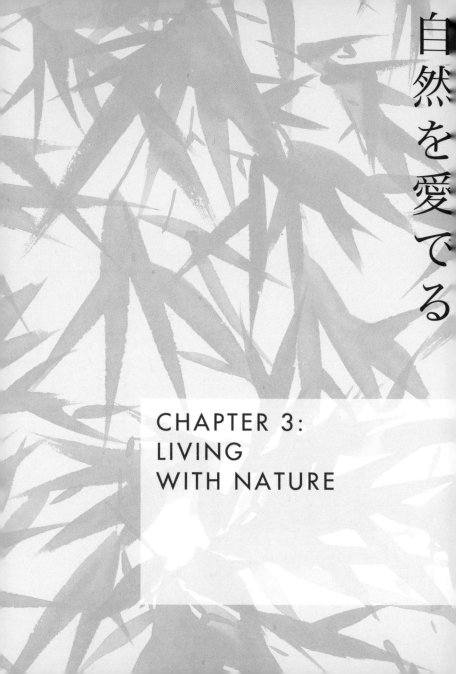

自然を愛でる

CHAPTER 3:
LIVING
WITH NATURE

Millions of tourists are drawn to Japan every year by the lure of its natural treasures—mountains, volcanoes, hot springs, subtropical beaches, and some of the best snow in the world. There are reminders of nature and the seasons at every turn. People don't just look at nature, they live inside it, name themselves after it, feast on it, wear it, and are guided through life by it.

The nature connection

I'm shuffling along in my socks, trailing a Zen monk wearing samue (temple work clothes) and a small cloth cap. This monk from Zuihō-in Temple is a man of deep wisdom and scrolls of stories. I think I'm asking too many questions for such a quiet place, but he's so fascinating I can't help myself. I have booked an appointment to sit inside Taian, a replica of Sen no Rikyū's original teahouse, built in honor of the four-hundredth anniversary of his death. We have paused for a moment to admire a simple sand garden from the wooden veranda, when the monk notices two other temple visitors just around the corner.

One is a manicured guy with sharp clothes but tired eyes, carrying a silver-studded tote bag. Transplanted from the bustle and bright lights of Tōkyō by the bullet train in just a few hours to this quiet temple in Kyōto, he looks disoriented. The monk steps forward to talk to him.

"Oi, have you come from Ginza?" he asks in a surprisingly familiar tone.

"No, Akasaka," blurts the man with the bloodshot eyes, looking to his girlfriend as if for confirmation. She looks exhausted, too.

"What's your job?" the monk wants to know.

"I work in commercial communications," the visitor replies, clearly unsure as to why he is having a career conversation with a Zen monk in a sand garden.

"Huh? What's that? You mean ads? Selling stuff?"

"Umm . . . yes," says the man from Tōkyō, looking down at his stockinged feet uncomfortably.

It's pretty obvious what the monk thinks of this career choice. It's less a judgment than a show of pity for this guy, who clearly works late into the night and probably survives on a diet of energy drinks and midnight rāmen.

"I think spending time in a temple is going to do you good," says the monk. And then to me, "Do you mind?"

I had made a solo reservation to view the place but this felt like a gathering of three weary travelers who could do with some tearoom serenity.

"Of course not," I reply.

And so the monk takes us all under his wing and flies us into Taian, the smallest tearoom I have ever seen. Made solely from individually selected pieces of wood, the tiny building is exquisite. Inside, hazy sunbeams filter through the paper-covered windows and hover in the air, searching in vain for dust motes. The corners are dark, yet the hanging scroll seems to glow in the tokonoma *alcove.*

In this intimate space, representing hundreds of years of culture and history, I break the silence to ask about wabi sabi.

The monk pauses for a moment, tilts his head, and offers this: "Wabi sabi is naturalness; it's about things in their natural, most authentic state. That's all."

The man from Tōkyō nods his head slowly, recognition dawning on his face. "Naruhodo," he says. "I see." And then, "How come I had to travel all this way, and wait all these years, and have a foreigner ask that question, before I could know the answer?"

The Japanese love of nature

The monk's thoughts notwithstanding, it is unexpectedly challenging to explain the connection between *wabi sabi* and nature. It's like trying to see something under a microscope, but getting up so close that it's actually blurry. A *wabi sabi* worldview is one predicated on the fundamental truths of nature and the cycle of life. *Wabi sabi* is born of a people whose traditional view of nature is that they are part of, not separate from, it. And yet because *wabi sabi* and nature are so closely related, we get this blurred view when trying to put words to that connection. To see it more clearly, we have to pull away a little, refocus our microscope and adjust our eyes.

According to the Cambridge English dictionary, nature is "all the animals, plants, rocks, etc. in the world and all the features, forces, and processes that happen or exist independently of people, such as the weather, the sea, mountains, the production of young animals or plants, and growth" and "the force that is responsible for physical life and that is sometimes spoken of as a person."[1] The main definition given in *Kōjien*, the Japanese equivalent of this dictionary, simply states: "Things as they are."[2]

At its essence, the experience of *wabi sabi* is an intuitive response to beauty that reflects the true nature of things as they are. That is, a beauty that reminds us that everything is impermanent, imperfect, and incomplete. This experience of *wabi sabi* is often felt in the presence of natural materials, which is why spending time in nature can be such a powerful experience. It reminds us that we are part of something miraculous. By momentarily lifting us out of the fog of to-do lists, chores, and overwhelming tasks, *wabi sabi* holds up a mirror to life's magnificence—and in that mirror, we get a glimpse of ourselves.

The forest does not care what your hair looks like. The mountains don't move for any job title. The rivers keep running, regardless of your social-media following, your salary, or your popularity. The flowers keep on blooming, whether or not you make mistakes. Nature just is, and welcomes you, just as you are.

Our capacity to experience *wabi sabi* reconnects us to these truths, which allow us to feel, in the moment, unconditionally accepted.

The influence of nature on literature, art, and culture

When I consulted with a Japanese professor on the translation of "living with nature," they suggested *shizen o mederu* (自然を愛でる), which actually means "loving nature."

This endemic love of nature, which has ancient roots in religion, has heavily influenced the arts and literature over the centuries. Still today, nature influences the rhythms and rituals of daily life, and particular attention is paid to the changing seasons in Japan.

As a teenager, I had a haiku poem by Matsuo Bashō pinned on my bedroom wall. It read: "The first Winter rains. From now on my name shall be Traveler."[3] In just a few words, the gifted poet captured all my ideas about adventure and discovery out in the big, wide, and wild world outside my bedroom door, while simultaneously transporting me to a cold, wet day in seventeenth-century Japan.

The Tale of Genji, the world's first novel, written a millennium ago by Murasaki Shikibu, is filled with references to nature and the changing seasons. Likewise, *The Pillow Book*, written at a similar time by Sei Shōnagon, opened with the classic line "*Haru wa akebono*" ("In spring, the dawn").[4] The whole opening section of this famous Heian-period court journal goes into detail about the writer's favorite parts of each season. There are many more nature references throughout *The Pillow Book,* which remains a classic ten centuries later.

The Japanese have been writing about nature and the seasons for as long as they have been writing.

Japanese nature writing emphasizes not just a sense of place but also, crucially, a sense of time. This is evoked by seasonal references or implications, and through observations of impermanence. This impermanence is expressed in two ways—through the absence of something that was but is no longer, and through the notion of transience, in the sense of something that is but will soon no longer be.

One of Japan's most influential poets, Fujiwara no Teika (1162–1241), often wrote about the seasons in this way, weaving together nature and literature with heavy vines of emotion. From the woodblock prints of Hokusai to the contemporary films of Studio Ghibli's Hayao Miyazaki, nature is everywhere in Japanese art, too.

Japanese architecture is also heavily influenced by nature, as discussed in chapter 2. Cultivated nature plays an important role, too, central as it is to many traditional aspects of Japanese culture—in ikebana (flower arranging), the nurturing of bonsai, the tea ceremony, and so on. One of the country's native instruments, the *shakuhachi*, is a flute made from bamboo. In the hands of a skilled player, it can replicate many sounds of nature, from rushing water and eerie winds to honking geese and pouring rain.

Nature in language

Nature-related words are frequently used in both people's names and place-names. A quick scan of a map of Japan will reveal the likes of Akita (Autumn Rice Paddy), Chiba (One Thousand Leaves), and Kagawa (Fragrant River).

Some of the most popular boys' names in recent years include Asahi (朝陽, Morning Sun) and Haru (晴, Fine Weather), while popular girls' names include Aoi (葵, Hollyhock), An (杏, Apricot), and Mio (美桜, Beautiful Cherry Blossom).[5] And it's not just first names. In the top ten most popular family names in Japan we find Kobayashi (小林, Small Forest) and Yamamoto (山本, Mountain Origin).[6]

There are beautiful words for particular happenings in nature, such as *komorebi* (木漏れ日), which describes sunlight filtering through the trees, dappling the earth below. *Kogarashi* (木枯し) expresses a particular kind of winter wind. And there are at least fifty ways to describe rain in the Japanese language. Onomatopoeia is used extensively, including to convey sounds related to nature. *Zāzā* describes rain pouring down heavily, *kopokopo* suggests the gentle bubbling of water, and *hyūhyū* is the sound of a whooshing wind.

There are entire almanacs of seasonal words to use in poetry, and guides to writing letters and emails with season-specific greetings. A recent missive from a male Japanese friend began:

Hello, Beth,

How are you?
The narcissi started to bloom yesterday, and the cherry blossom is on its way. We had Chinese chives from the garden for breakfast this morning. They tasted delicious, and show us that spring has come . . .

The most beautiful thing about notes that open in this way is their power to reveal a momentary window into the writer's life, through the details of the seasons they are experiencing at the time. In a few lines, they can transport you to the warmth of a patch of sunlight beneath a plum tree or legs tucked under a *kotatsu* (heated table) eating *mikan* (satsumas), while the snow falls softly outside.

The rhythm of the seasons

Creating our own seasonal traditions can be a wonderful way to honor the rhythms of nature and notice the passage of time in our own lives.

One of my favorite memories of life in rural Japan was the time my elderly neighbor Sakamoto-*banchan* ("Grandmother Sakamoto" in the local dialect), a delightful lady in her late eighties, corralled me into helping her make *hoshi-gaki* (dried persimmons). She taught me that after peeling the firm fruits, you tie the stalks together with a long piece of string and hang them over a bamboo pole. Then you leave them to dry. For the first week, you don't touch them, but then you give them regular gentle massages over the next three weeks or so. This draws the fructose to the surface, so they end up looking like they have been dipped in sugar. Tasting note: *Hoshi-gaki* are delicious with green tea.

Ever since she was a little girl, every year for eight decades, Sakamoto-*banchan* had carried out this ritual of food preparation. To her, *hoshi-gaki were* autumn.

The *wabi sabi* connection

So how does all this connect to *wabi sabi*? In a subtle, beautiful, *komorebi*-sunshine-filtering-through-the-leaves kind of way.

Each ray of natural inspiration is a reminder to notice and appreciate what is here now in all its ephemeral beauty. If you visit Japan, you will soon realize how the four main seasons of spring, summer, autumn, and winter[7] are woven into the fabric of everyday life: spring brings cherry blossom and *hanami* (flower-viewing) parties, summer offers festivals and kimono-clad strolls along the river in search of fireflies; autumn welcomes moon viewing and *momiji* (maple) leaves, especially memorable when lit up at night; and winter ushers in the quiet beauty of snow. There is evidence of the seasons in the tiniest of details, from food to decoration, from clothing to festivals.

I suspect that the importance of these observances, the rituals and traditions and the thousands of tiny reminders in daily life, are the reason that *wabi sabi* is so deeply embedded in the hearts of the Japanese people.

Marking time

Japanese people have paid close attention to the seasons since ancient times. According to the classical Japanese calendar, there are in fact twenty-four small seasons known as *sekki* (節季), each lasting around fifteen days, and seventy-two microseasons known as *kō* (候), each lasting around five days.[8] The calendar was originally adopted from China in AD 862 and eventually reformed to suit the local climate (particularly around Kyōto) by court astronomer Shibukawa Shunkai in 1684.[9] Each of these sub seasons and microseasons has a name, which paints an evocative picture of what is going on in the natural world at that particular time.

A quick tour of the year with some of my favorite microseason names would include: "East wind melts the ice," "Nightingales sing," "Mist starts to hover," "Cherry blossoms open," "Silkworms hatch," "Grain ripens," "Hot winds arrive," "Earth is steaming wet," "Blanket fog descends," "Rice ripens," "Swallows leave," "First frost," and "North wind rattles the leaves."[10]

The seasons are a kind of *wabi sabi* metronome, a steady call back to the present, to noticing, savoring, and treasuring.

QUESTIONS TO HELP YOU TUNE IN TO NATURE

Whatever time of year, wherever in the world you are, you can use the prompts below to help you notice more about what is going on in your immediate surroundings. Try to use all your senses and look for the details. If you return to this over the course of a year, you'll discover how tracking the seasons can change the way you see the world.

1. What is the weather like? Consider water, wind, sun, and any conditions specific to where you are.
2. What is the light like?
3. What is the night sky like?
4. What plants and flowers are emerging? Blooming? Fading? Hiding?
5. What animals have you noticed recently?
6. What ingredients are in season right now?

7. What have you been wearing when you go outdoors lately?
8. What seasonal colors have you noticed lately?
9. What seasonal sounds have you noticed lately?
10. What seasonal smells have you noticed lately?
11. What seasonal textures have you noticed lately?
12. How do you feel? What is your mood?
13. How is your health? How are your energy levels?
14. What self-care do you need to be practicing right now? How could you yield to the season?
15. What traditions or observances have you celebrated recently?
16. Dig into memory. What nature-related or seasonal traditions did you grow up with, either in your own home or in your community? How could you bring an element of those traditions into your life now?
17. How could you mark this particular season in some gentle way?

Tuning in to your natural rhythm

The Japanese expression *ichiyō ochite tenka no aki o shiru* (一葉落ちて天下の秋を知る) tells us that "with the fall of a single leaf we know that autumn is here." As a proverb, it is used in the context of recognizing imminent change. The Japanese see the seasons as signposts, visible reminders of our own natural rhythms.

In modern life, these often get disrupted, as we extend our days with strong artificial light, interrupt our sensitive biorhythms with blue lights from our electronic devices, and push ourselves to be highly productive just because it's another weekday. We push on, regardless of whether our body is trying to tell us it's time to hibernate or get outside for some summer sunshine—and then we wonder why we get sick.

The seasons are a regular reminder that we don't need to push all the time. Every push needs a pull. Every expansion needs a contraction. Every effort needs a rest. There are times for creating and times for seeking inspiration. Times for noise and times for silence. Times to focus and times to dream. Ebb and flow. Wax and wane. There are those contrasts again. *Wabi sabi* invites you to tune in to your natural rhythm, in this season of your life, in this season of the year, in this moment of your day.

Lessons from the fire festival

Normally, the tiny village of Kurama in the north of Kyōto is a peaceful place where visitors relax in the natural hot spring or follow the shrine trail far on up the mountain. But today is different. Today is the annual Hi-Matsuri (fire festival) and the stories of blazing torches and glowing skies have lured others, too. Lots of others. The streets are alive as dusk falls and the darkness creeps in.

The chanting has begun. Stamping follows. Men clothed in little more than G-strings and leafy miniskirts start pacing the streets, slowly at first, getting accustomed to the weight of the fifteen-foot torch on their shoulders. Small children clutch their own burning brands, following in their fathers' footsteps, proud smiles revealed by the dancing flames of two hundred and fifty pine torches.

The soft chant increases in volume and intensity until the words become a war cry filling the raw night air. Through the streets they march, past the crowds and up the front steps of the Shintō shrine Yuki-jinja, on a mission intended to guide the kami *(spirits or gods) on their way.*

Festivals like this have been celebrated since ancient times and still take place all year round across Japan. Many have strong religious connections. Others relate to agriculture, the seasons, or the marking of different stages of life. Virtually all of them are tied to nature or the cycle of life in some way.

The way of the *kami*

We have mentioned the influence of Buddhism, but we must also consider the influence of Shintō, Japan's indigenous religious tradition. Meaning "The Way of the *Kami*," Shintō is "intimately connected with the agricultural cycle and a sense of sacredness of the natural world,"[11] and centers around the worship of *kami* (spirits or gods). *Kami* can be found in both animate and inanimate objects, from mountains and streams to animals and rocks.

In the words of now retired Shintō grand master Motohisa Yamakage: "As part of their everyday lives, and without recourse to complex philosophy, the Japanese people have loved and revered nature as a gift from Kami since ancient times."[12]

Dr. Sokyō Ono, Shintō scholar and author of *Shintō: The Kami Way,* said:

> Shrine worship is closely associated with a keen sense of the beautiful, a mystic sense of nature which plays an important part in leading the mind of man from the mundane to the higher and deeper world of the divine and in transforming his life into an experience of living with the kami. No amount of artificial beauty is an adequate substitute for the beauty of nature.[13]

Lessons from the Yamabushi

I have long been fascinated by the Yamabushi, mountain-based ascetic hermits who make their home in the Dewa Sanzan (three sacred mountains) area of Yamagata Prefecture, where I used to live. When out hiking on Mount Haguro, I would occasionally catch a glimpse of them heading off silently on a mountain retreat, in their white robes, carrying *horagai* conch trumpets. The religion of the Yamabushi is called *Shugendō*, often described as an integration of aspects of Buddhism, Shintō, and Taoism.

For many years, it has been something of a rite of passage for city dwellers to undergo intense training and a sacred pilgrimage with the Yamabushi, which includes meditating beneath an ice-cold waterfall. Recently, this training has been opened up to non-Japanese people.[14]

Master Hoshino, the thirteenth-generation Yamabushi who leads the program, told me, "People always ask me the meaning of Yamabushi training. It's the philosophy of putting yourself in nature and thinking about what you feel. First, we experience. Then we reflect. There are things that can't be learned without being directly experienced. On the mountain, the mountain is the teacher."

The core philosophy of Yamabushi training is the single word *uketamō* (受けたもう), which means "I humbly accept." It is a powerful invitation to openness and mindfulness. This is a wonderful mantra for any time spent in nature, when we want to invite nature to be our teacher.

Lessons from the forest

It's not often I find myself lying faceup on a snow-covered forest floor, tracking bird flight while listening for the distant sound of water. Above me, the trees are silhouetted against a sky the color of stonewashed jeans, the tips of the smaller branches silvered by the late-winter sun.

I am in Takashima, a small town on the edge of Lake Biwa, treating myself to the grounding experience of shinrin-yoku *(森林浴, forest bathing)—a term coined in 1982 by the director general of Japan's*

agriculture, forestry, and fisheries agency, Tomohide Akiyama. A rel-
atively new therapy, originating in Japan, it has now been scientifically
proven to confirm something we have always known in our bones: trees
can make us well.

As our lives become increasingly fast-paced and sanitized, many of us are feeling disconnected from nature and from ourselves, as if something important is missing. People have long understood that spending time in nature, and specifically among trees in a forest, has a calming effect, but it is only in the past decade or so that consistent peer-reviewed scientific results have added weight to the idea of it as a preventive medicine. This has subsequently led to use of the term "forest therapy." Results point to increased mental wellness, boosted immune systems, and reduced stress levels, heart rate, and blood pressure.[15]

These effects are due not only to the calm atmosphere and gentle exercise, but also to actual interactions with the trees. One piece of research found that after a forest-bathing trip, subjects had significantly higher numbers of so-called natural killer (NK) cells, a type of lymphocyte that boosts the immune system's defenses against viruses and cancers—an effect that lasted for seven days after the experience. Further studies have suggested that the immune boost was, at least in part, a result of exposure to phytoncides, a substance emitted by plants and trees.[16]

Back in the forest, home to deer, monkeys, wild boar, and bears, March
has arrived, but the cold season lingers; the trees are still dark and bare.
Birds' nests are easier to see when there is no leaf coverage. I watch a
couple of feathered friends, nuthatches perhaps, hop from branch to branch
in playful chase, and delight in having nowhere else to be.

Our guide, Mr. Shimizu, is an energetic retiree with fantastic knowl-
edge of the local flora and fauna. Head to toe in red, with a bottle of green
tea hanging from his belt, he carries a stethoscope around his neck, for

listening to water, of course. He is one of hundreds of certified forest therapy guides working at official sites across Japan.

Shimizu-san has seen this particular trail in every season and knows its secrets intimately. "Come and look at this moss," he calls, offering a magnifying glass. "And here, see how the snow has melted around the trunks of these beech trees? That's their energy at work." He invites us to go slowly, use all our senses, and notice the details of the world alive all around us.

Our therapy session had begun a couple of hours earlier. First, we washed our hands in a small stream, feeling the coolness of the water and listening to the gurgle as it fell over a low waterfall. A gentle hike took us to the base of a gully, from where a 180-degree turn offered a view of distant fields and mountains. There, we stopped for water and roasted almonds, before our first silent exercise. We each had to pick a direction and look first to the far distance, then the middle distance, then up close, to see how the same view changed, depending on what we focused on.

In other forest-therapy sessions, you might hear flute music, spend time in a hammock to soak in the healing power of the trees, meditate, or go barefoot to sense different surfaces beneath your feet. It depends on the location, the guide, and the season.

"It is clear that our bodies still recognize nature as our home, which is important to consider as increasing numbers of people are living in cities and urban environments," says Professor Yoshifumi Miyazaki, deputy director of the Centre for Environment Health and Field Sciences at Chiba University, who proposed the term "forest therapy" to describe *shinrin-yoku* supported by scientific evidence.[17]

His research has measured the direct benefits of forest therapy, which include an increase in those NK cells, known to fight tumors and infection; increased relaxation and reduced stress;

reduction in blood pressure after just fifteen minutes; and a general sense of well-being.

"It is not just forests that can have a beneficial effect on our well-being," Professor Miyazaki says. "Other natural stimuli, such as parks, flowers, *bonsai* and even pieces of wood have been shown to reduce stress, making these effects attainable for all of us, even city-dwellers."[18]

In the end, I was glad I had forced myself out from my cozy futon when the moon was still high in the sky, to catch an early train out to the forest. I left relaxed and rejuvenated, and slept like a baby that night.

Writing in *The Anatomy of Self*, a classic book looking into the Japanese character, psychiatrist Takeo Doi made the fascinating observation that Japanese people likely feel so fond of nature because when they are in it, they don't have to subscribe to any of society's rules: "They become one with nature so to speak.... From their viewpoint therefore they feel more human with nature than with humans."[19] I am pretty sure many non-Japanese people feel this way, too.

Natural wellness
There is great value in the scientific evidence that reassures skeptics of the benefits of spending time in forests, and official *shinrin-yoku* has encouraged large numbers of people into the woods, which is to be celebrated.

However, we should not be mistaken in thinking that you have to be on an official trail, with an official guide, to enjoy the healing power of the trees. I think we have a huge opportunity to take the principles of evidence-based forest therapy and let them loose in wilder areas. Walking. Hiking. Doing yoga among the trees. Climbing the trees. Embracing them.

Talking to them. Sitting with our backs to the trees writing in our journals.

There is a lovely phrase in Japanese, *kachō fūgetsu* (花鳥風月). It literally means "flower-bird-wind-moon." It refers to contemplating the beauty of nature. This kind of contemplation can prompt reflection on our own inner nature and remind us of our role as part of a magnificent whole, which puts everything in perspective.

The forest invites us to open our hearts and listen.

My hope for forest bathing is that it becomes like yoga—a practice that is worth learning from a trained teacher but can also be done alone or in a small group, away from too much structure and equipment and rules. Just you and the trees—or maybe you, the trees, and your yoga mat—finding your own rhythm and deepening your connection with nature.

The medicine of the forest is far more than a contemporary wellness trend. People have lived in forests since ancient times. Nature is in our blood. It's in our bones. It's in our very human spirit. It is the haunting call of the mountains and the swirling pull of the sea; the whispering of the wind and the secrets in the trees.

To me, forest bathing is not about doing something new; it's about something we know deep down, but that many of us have forgotten. When you spend time in a gentle forest and experience moments of mindfulness among the trees, you feel held, supported, transported. It's like coming back to an old friend, who will pull you in close and whisper secrets in your ear if only you'll show up at their door.

In the modern world, we spend so much of our time shut up in sanitized boxes—in our homes, our cars, our offices. Taking time to step out of those boxes and get close to the wild outdoors sharpens our senses and reminds us of the preciousness of life. We sometimes need everything to be stripped away to reveal the true beauty. We need the simplicity to remind us that life isn't all about accumulating stuff. And we need the birdsong and big skies to remind us that we are part of nature. Wildness is a part of who we are.

Top tips for forest bathing

Here are some tips for forest bathing among trees near you. Why not take a copy of this list with you the next time you go for a woodland adventure:

- Walk slowly. Now slow your pace by half. And by half again.
- Be present. Keep your phone in your pocket.
- Use all your senses to explore your environment. Notice the feel of the ground under your feet, the taste of the air, the wind in the trees, the light and the shadows. Look up, down, and all around.
- Cup your hands behind your ears to capture more sounds of the forest. What can you hear? Where is the sound coming from? Is it low down or high up? Is it near or far?
- Touch things. Notice how different bark, branches, and leaves feel.
- Notice where things are in their life cycle. What is emerging? What is growing? What is fading?
- Breathe deeply. What can you smell?
- Watch the sky. Look for movement. Count colors. How many shades of one color can you see? Stay watching long enough to notice changes.
- If you can identify what is safe to eat, taste a berry or a leaf slowly, and with gratitude.
- Pick up a fallen gift of the forest and look at it closely. What can you see?

- Spend some time in silence, even if you are in a group. In fact, especially if you are in a group. Try meditating, stretching, or just sitting with your back against a tree.
- Lie in a hammock between two trees. Ask the trees' permission before you set up camp.
- Take off your shoes and feel the earth beneath your feet or dip your toes in a stream.
- Notice how you feel when you are held by the forest. Don't rush. Linger as long as you can.
- Find a particular spot you are drawn to and spend time there. Name it. Make up a story about it. Come back on another day, in another season, and see what has changed.

While taking a moment in nature, ask yourself these questions:

- How do you feel when you are being held by the forest?
- What stories of the land rise up to greet you as you stretch your arms wide and open your heart?
- What secrets might you want to share with the running river or the wise old tree?
- What wishes will you scatter in the woods like fallen leaves, to be carried on the wind to a place you cannot know?
- What promise do you make to yourself, on this day, in this place?

Note: Please be sure to take the usual safety precautions when going into the forest. And if you cannot get to a cluster of trees near you right now, try putting cypress or cedar oil in your diffuser or bring some plants into your home. (See chapter 2 for other ideas on how to bring nature indoors.)

Nurturing a harmonious relationship

On a recent hike with some Japanese friends, we came to an outcrop of rock with a fallen log, perfect for a sit-down and some freshly brewed *kuromoji-cha* (spicewood tea). It was a new flavor for me, a little spicy at first, but then sweet. Delicious. In between sipping our drinks, making a miniature snowman, and pointing out tiny buds promising spring, we talked about how and why we love nature.

We also had a tricky conversation about the way so much of Japanese nature has been destroyed so rapidly in the past century or so. Although quintessential images of Japan often include images of nature, such as vast swathes of cherry blossom or the iconic peak of Mount Fuji, it's no secret that much of Japan's natural landscape and wildlife have been decimated by the acceleration of industrialization since the 1868 Meiji Restoration[20] and the rise to economic power in the latter half of the twentieth century.

The overriding sense I got from the group was that they do feel part of nature, not separated from it, but they fear that many people have lost some of that sense of connection in the rush for economic progress. The truth is, much of the environment that inspired the likes of Bashō (1644–94) and Hokusai (1760–1849) is either gone or hard to photograph these days without a power line or building featuring in the foreground. My friends recognized that the well-documented Japanese love of nature seems incongruent with the vast amounts of concrete in Japan's urban jungles and all the cables crisscrossing the sky.

This sense of a weakening connection with nature has been echoed by film director Hayao Miyazaki in many of his famous anime (animated films). His films express the Shintō view that there is continuity between man and nature, and he has used his films to address the issues that arise when humanity separates from nature, whether by trying to control or destroy it.

This major challenge of our times requires us to get back to nature, not move further away from it.

The impermanence of awe

It is a gray January morning and I am en route to the Bodleian Japanese Library in Oxford to do some research for this book when I look up to see not one but two rainbows in the sky. I am rooted to the spot, gazing in awe at this gift, the like of which I have never seen. As I watch, I can see it changing, now stronger, now fading. A teenage boy walks in my direction with his head down and almost bumps into me, so invested is he in the phone in his hand. "Look," I say, tapping his arm and pointing to the sky, unable to contain myself. "Wow," he says, and turns to stand beside me, two strangers sharing the perfect moment of a double rainbow. Two minutes later it is gone.

Nature is the home of miracles. Complex growth, stories of resilience, ephemeral beauty emerging and evaporating. When we take the time to stop and look, each one of these gifts reminds us to pay attention to the fleeting beauty of our own lives.

WABI SABI–INSPIRED WISDOM
FOR LIVING WITH NATURE

- *Nature reminds us of the transience of our own lives.*
- *Paying attention to the passing of the seasons is a way to stay present.*
- *The rhythms of nature remind us to tune in to our own natural rhythms, so we know when to surge forth and when to relax.*

TRY IT: PONDERING

Spend some time in nature contemplating:

❋   The transience of life

❋   The beauty in the light and the darkness

❋   The tiny details and the vast horizon

❋   The seasonal clues and gifts

❋   The sensual experience of the weather

What do you notice? When you really listen, what is it telling you?

吾唯足知

CHAPTER 4:
ACCEPTANCE +
LETTING GO

There are two ways to translate a sentence between English and Japanese. One is *chokuyaku*—a direct translation of the actual words; the other is *iyaku*, a contextual translation of the meaning. The literal *chokuyaku* may be considered more "perfect," in terms of translating every part of the sentence, but it doesn't take into account the context of its reception, just as an idea of a "perfect life" doesn't take into account the context of our own complex and challenging reality. It's often the *iyaku*—the seemingly "imperfect"

Everything is impermanent, imperfect, and incomplete.

version—that is infinitely more powerful, graceful, and valuable, giving the more authentic translation, just as the "imperfect life" is the authentic way of living.

One of the core teachings of *wabi sabi* is the acceptance of the true nature of life: everything is impermanent, imperfect, and incomplete.

In this chapter, we are going to look at that acceptance in relation to ourselves, and in relation to our past, present, and future. By the end, I hope you will feel a shift, having experienced the release of tension and the surge in personal power that comes with letting go of "perfect" and accepting what is, standing on fresh ground with this new perspective.

Things change. That's life.

Every time I go to Kyōto, it is familiar yet different. Buildings have gone up, buildings have come down. New shops have appeared, others have vanished. One favorite café has given way to another. Over the years, this city has been altered by war and earthquakes, fires and tourism. And, of course, the changing seasons are a part of daily life here, a visual and emotional reminder of the passage of time.

Recently, I met up with an old friend in Tōkyō who I hadn't seen in more than a decade. On seeing each other we both squealed, "You haven't changed a bit!" although, in truth, of course we had both changed in so many ways. Since we last got together I had gotten married, had two children, built a business, and moved more times than I care to remember. She had spent time abroad, switched careers, battled an illness, lost a parent, and learned a new language. . . . Each of these formative experiences has shaped us, sometimes a little, sometimes a lot.

Our lives, relationships, careers, health, finances, attitudes, interests, capabilities, responsibilities, and opportunities are changing all the time. Sometimes the change is significant or fast, and you feel it as clearly as a rushing wind. Other times the change will be minor or slow, like a daffodil raising its head to the sun and you have to pay close attention to see it.

Nowhere ever stays completely still. And neither do we. *Wabi sabi* teaches us that dynamic transience is the natural state of all things. And as change is inevitable, trying to hold on to the past or the present is pointless and stressful.

Over the many years I have spent supporting people through major life transitions, I have noticed how vastly different our attitudes toward change can be. At one end of the spectrum are those who are terrified of it and will do absolutely anything within their power to hold on to the status quo, even when they don't actually like it. At the other end are those who embrace change as an escape mechanism, often habitually, so that as soon as things start to get difficult, they jump to something else, often later chastising themselves for never sticking to anything. And there are many in the middle who recognize the need to change and genuinely want to embrace it, but are stalled by fear. I wonder where you sit on that continuum?

I was talking to a friend about the idea of transience over red rice and *niimono* (simmered vegetables) at his home in a rural suburb of Tōkyō. He gestured toward his garden, where a small bamboo forest stood and said:

> You can see change happening right there. The bamboo is growing all the time, and is also sensitive to its dynamic environment. It's firmly rooted but flexible. When the wind blows, the bamboo doesn't resist; it lets go and moves with it. And still the forest grows. Think of the buildings in this earthquake-prone country. The ones that survive the shaking are those that can move when the trembling begins.

Flexibility is strength. Be like the bamboo.

I think I just had a Mr. Miyagi moment.

Stability can make us feel safe, but it is a precarious stability that is built on the misguided assumption that things won't change, because everything does. When a sudden change comes from an external source—a layoff, a loss, an affair, an illness, for example—the shock is considerable. Rigidity actually makes us vulnerable to that. If it hits us when we are desperately trying to hang on to what we know, it can knock us flat. But if we are accepting of what is happening (not necessarily happy about it or condoning it, but realistic about the fact that it is going on), we may be blown about but not completely knocked off balance, and we can recover sooner.

Accepting the past

It is so easy to spend time caught up in the past, lost in nostalgia, heavy with regret, chastising yourself for not having made different choices or blaming someone else. Back then, you didn't know all you know now. You didn't have the same resources, environment, or responsibilities. Perhaps you didn't have the same outlook, self-awareness, courage, or support. Or maybe you look back on the past as the golden years, when things were easier and you were more this or more that. But here's the thing: the past is no longer here. Whatever happened, the good and the bad, it is gone.

Whatever it is that keeps pulling you back, take a moment to make peace with it, then let it go. This sounds hard, but it can be as simple as deciding to do it. Write it out. Speak to a professional if you need to or talk to a friend. Then pick a day—like your birthday, or the turn of a season, or the new year, or the next Tuesday—and make it the day you leave that particular thing in the past. It is only you that keeps paying it attention.

Wabi sabi teaches us to accept that the past was then, and it was what it was. This is now, and it is what it is. Your life is happening right here, and every day is the beginning of the rest of it.

Accepting the present

Acceptance is alignment with the truth of the present moment. In this present moment, what is true about your life? You are holding this book, opening yourself up to ideas from another culture. Perhaps you are drinking a cup of your favorite tea or you keep getting distracted by a fly buzzing around the room.

Maybe your window is open and you can hear cars going past. Or the sun is casting shadows across your desk. Perhaps you are at the hairdresser's, getting ready for a special night out. Or you have just come back to this page after an inspiring conversation, or a big argument, or some surprising news. Maybe you are reading this on the bus or in your kitchen with half an eye on the oven to see if your pie is baked.

I wonder if you are hot or cold or just right? If you can smell cooking or the garden or the impending rain. Do you have music playing? Is the clock ticking? Are you soaking in the tub listening to the sound of your own breathing?

Take a moment to think about the facts of your life in this exact moment. This moment is the one you are living right now. You cannot extend it forever. At some point the pie will be done, the bathwater will go cold, the night will close in. Accepting that we cannot hold on to or control the status quo is a powerful lesson from *wabi sabi*, reminding us to treasure the good we have right now, and know that the bad will pass.

Any time you feel stressed or worried, upset, lost, or lonely, anchor yourself in the facts of now. Notice what's going on in your body and what's going on around you. Feel what you are feeling. Know that this is just a moment and soon it will give way to another.

Any time you are feeling overwhelmed, try to accept that what is possible in the present is limited. You can only do what you can do. This is not a shutting off of possibilities but rather a recognition of your own capacity, so you can stop expecting impossible things of yourself and give yourself a break.

Any time you recognize a moment of true joy, soak it all up. Anchor yourself to the sights, sounds, and smells of right there and then, so they can transform into a precious memory when the moment has passed, which it will.

Lessons from Ryōan-ji

I distinctly remember the day I first saw the famous stone *tsukubai* (washbasin) in the grounds of Ryōan-ji temple in Kyōto.

I am nineteen years old, and I have stopped off at this temple on my way home from language school. Around the back of the main building from the famous raked-sand garden lies an unassuming tsukubai, *tucked into an enclave of mossy rocks and greenery. But I can tell by the attention it is attracting that this is no ordinary washbasin. Each of the temple visitors stops to look, crouch down to pick up the bamboo ladle, scoop up some water, and wash their hands. One at a time they pause for thought. Many take photos. It is clearly more than a ritual cleansing and I want to know what all the fuss is about.*

Up close, I see four characters set around a central square section, which holds the water. Still quite new to the language, I am proud that I can recognize the character at the top, which represents the number five. But I cannot read the others and am puzzled by what is drawing the visitors in. Summoning up courage, I approach one of the monks, point to the tsukubai, *and ask what it means.*

He says, "Ware tada taru o shiru." *None of these words means "five" so I am still none the wiser. I draw a picture of it and go home to consult my dictionary and my host mother.*

Eventually, I figure out that the four characters don't mean much individually, but when you combine each with the central square 口, they become the four characters 吾 唯 足 知, which is the "ware tada taru o shiru" the monk mentioned. A direct translation would be something like "I only know plenty." A more poetic rendition might be "Rich is the person who is content with what they have," or "I have everything I need."

We have everything we need.

The message has been there all along. This is wisdom we carry inside us. Recognition of what we already have is the key to contentment. We just have to accept it, trust it, and embrace it.

What do we mean by perfect?

The "perfect life" that we are sold over and over is the one we see in ads—a predictable, stylized version of the human experience that eliminates the dimension of difficult emotion and hard-earned experience. It's often a shiny-haired, perfectly manicured, wrinkle-free picture of bliss, running on a beach, sitting in a beautiful home, or laughing with a bunch of equally shiny-haired, perfectly manicured, wrinkle-free friends. Or it is the Instagram feed of the perfectly styled home, perfectly behaved children, or perfectly honed body.

If only we owned the latest handbag or car or gym member-ship, our lives would be perfect, too. What we forget is that the ads are showing manufactured moments in a movie-set life and the stylized social-media streams are carefully curated brand stories, not real life itself.

Either that or the marketing professionals cleverly remind us why our lives are hard, in a way that makes us feel like things being hard is somehow wrong. Like we are doing life wrong.

We all know this. Yet, even so, we rack up the debt and fill up our homes and schedules and minds in the pursuit of the per-fect version that has sucked us in, instead of taking the time to figure out what really matters to us. It's like trying to get instant nourishment from the plastic bowl of rāmen in the window of a noodle shop instead of finding the courage to step inside, take a seat at the bar, order in our best Japanese accent, and show a little patience while the chef works their magic, so we can partake of the real thing.

As a monk[1] told me over green tea, with a gentle smile on his face:

Living is suffering. Getting sick is suffering. Growing old is suffering. Dying is suffering. We cannot avoid any of these things. When we try to resist them, we just compound the suffering and delay our ability to respond. If, instead, you can embrace the actuality of what is going on, then you can flow with life. People think Zen is all about calmness and tran-quility and living in some blissed-out state of good vibes. But actually it's about how you face your challenges: unhappiness, loneliness, worry, difficult emotions. It's about learning to deal with what life throws at you, and acceptance of actuality is central to that.

Acceptance is not about giving up or giving in. It's about surrendering to the truth of what is happening and then playing an active role in deciding what happens next. For example, if you are sick, it's about recognizing that you are sick, accepting that you are not at full capacity, giving yourself permission to slow down in order to heal, and asking for help when you need it rather than powering on through.

Surrendering to the truth of suffering in any area of your life allows you to proactively decide your next steps, with clarity, compassion, and a degree of ease. This teaching is many centuries old. And yet we still resist it.

There are many ways in which we inadvertently use perfection—and perfectionism—to stop us from embracing life:

- As a defense mechanism
- As a stalling tactic
- As an excuse
- As a form of control
- As a weapon
- As a judgment metric
- As a mask for a buried wound
- As an extreme response to criticism
- As a cloak to hide the truth

How many of these do you recognize? Did you realize the idea of perfection could be so harmful?

What do we mean by imperfect?

The "imperfection" that *wabi sabi* teaches us is based in the rules of nature. If everything is always changing, nothing can ever be absolutely complete. Therefore, nothing can ever be perfect, as perfection is a state of completeness.

We often use the word "imperfection" to describe a state that falls short of a perfection we have come to perceive as ideal, whether that is in objects or in ourselves, in looks, bank balance, achievements, or elsewhere in our lives. Any thesaurus will readily offer you a host of antonyms for "perfect," including flawed, corrupt, inferior, second-rate, inept, unsophisticated, broken, and bad. No wonder we see the opposite of perfect as a negative.

In order to eliminate the negativity around imperfection, we have to reject its use as the opposite of this fictional ideal state and instead adopt imperfection as the ideal itself: imperfection is not a compromise.

Imperfection is not somewhere on the road to perfection, where we have to stop because we've run out of gas. Imperfection is a snapshot of our journeys of growth and living at a particular moment in time. We've been so busy trying to get the car up the hill that we have forgotten to turn around and look out over the beauty of all that lies around us right now.

Imperfection is not a compromise.

We need to trust and accept and be willing to say: I don't know it all, but I don't need to know it all. I know enough. I don't have it all, but I don't need to have it all. I have enough. And I am not all things to all people, but I don't need to be all things to all people. I am doing my best to be all I can be to those who really matter. I am enough.

This does not mean having no goals or ambition and giving up, nor is it to suggest that striving for something is a bad thing. It's about getting really clear on why we want what we really want, outside of materialistic desires for the accumulation of stuff and the pressure of expectation from others. Let go of the push and the fight, the uphill battle to a place you don't need to get to. You can take all that energy you have been putting into the pursuit of perfection and pour it into living fully now. And once you start experiencing the world in this way, it looks and feels like a completely different place.

Revealing your imperfections

Accepting imperfection is one thing. Allowing others to see it is another. Yet that's often where we find common ground. Revealing our vulnerabilities, challenges, as-yet-unrealized dreams, and quirky joys opens a window into our hearts. People can see who we really are and they are drawn to connect.

Have you ever noticed how, when you find yourself in the presence of true beauty, your heart responds? It could be when you experience a person sharing their essence by speaking a gentle truth, a love poem whispered on the wind, a tiny hand in yours, or a moment of deep connection.

Your heart's response to beauty is the essence of *wabi sabi*.

When we are tuned in, our intuitive response comes faster than the logical analytical response, so we can feel something in our hearts before we have time to judge, criticize, compare, or get distracted. We can teach ourselves to experience others in this way, too. To meet someone with our hearts instead of just our minds, allowing our instinct and intuition to guide us beyond the judgment the mind creates based on what we see on the surface. And when we reveal our imperfections to others, we invite them to see us in a similar way.

I once cried onstage. Only once, but it happened. I was mortified. But the response from the audience was incredible. People didn't expect it. They could obviously sense that it was genuine feeling, although I wouldn't recommend it as a public-speaking technique. It does all sorts of strange things to your voice. But it allowed them to see my imperfections and to know that I was real. With nowhere to hide, I just let go and kept talking. The energy in the room shifted, as people opened their hearts to me, as I had opened mine to them. Afterward, the book-signing line was around the block, with many of those in the line crying, too, wanting to share their stories with me.

There is a tendency among self-help gurus to say things along these lines: "My life was a mess. One day I woke up to it. Now my life is amazing and perfect. You there, with your messed-up life, you can be like me and have an amazing, perfect life if you just read my book/take my course/join my workshop." But I don't buy it. We are all works in progress. Some of us happen to have had the opportunity to reflect, and perhaps have a platform from which to share what we are discovering as we go, but, in truth, we are all learning from one another. No one is in charge here. No one has all the answers. And anyone who pretends they do is either selling a false version of their story or heading for a wake-up call.

We can't possibly have it all together when we don't even know what all the pieces look like. And the sooner we realize this, the sooner we can start honoring ourselves and one another for the imperfect treasures that we are. We just have to trust that sometimes, when the head cannot find the answer, the heart knows the way.

Lessons from the bathhouse

I cannot imagine taking a bath in a public place in England, but visiting the *sento* is still a regular evening pastime for many people in Japan.

One snowy evening in Hida-Takayama, I venture around the corner from my rented place to Yutopia, paying ¥420 (about $3.77) for the privilege of an hour or two soaking in a large shared tub. After leaving all my clothes in a locker in the changing room, I head to the heat, naked but for a pair of plastic slippers.

It's steamy inside, and there are washing stations on two sides of the room. You have to crouch down and sit on a low stool, while you shower and wash your body with the aid of a plastic bucket. Someone thought it would be a good idea to put mirrors there. Still carrying fifteen pounds of baby weight I would like to have released a couple of years ago, I'm not sure I agree.

As I wash my hair, I can't help catching sight of some of the other women in the room. None of them is looking at me. They are all walking around straight-backed, with an air of quiet confidence, regardless of body shape, age, or any other defining factor that would render others among us self-conscious. There is an elderly lady soaking her aching limbs luxuriously in the Jacuzzi section. Two friends gossiping. A mother with her young child. I wonder what a difference it will make to that little girl's body confidence, having been brought up bathing in a public place like this.

For many years, girls in the West have been sold images of "perfection" that all look the same. Thankfully, this is starting to change, but we still have a long way to go. We are all heavily influenced by what we see, hear, and experience growing up, and we notice what our parents and other adults value through what they say, how they interact with others, and how they make decisions.

Suddenly, I notice how at ease I feel without my clothes, which is an unusual experience for this reserved Englishwoman. When those around me aren't paying my "flaws" any attention, neither am I. This evening in the bathhouse has taught me something important: my appreciation of my own imperfections is as much a gift to my daughters as it is to myself.

Choosing your role models carefully

The better we get at what we do, the more exposure we get to people who have done more, are "further ahead," have more "success." But as soon as we take our eyes off our own path and get lost in theirs, we miss the very experience of our own journey. It's like being on a train, traveling through a foreign country you have always wanted to visit, and then spending the whole trip watching a movie on your laptop. You miss the point and you miss the adventure.

There will always be some people who know more, have done more, or have more experience or knowledge than us in a particular field at a particular moment in time. We can choose to look at this as a reflection of a lack in ourselves or an opportunity for inspiration from them.

When the very people we admire and follow are the people who trigger a feeling of insufficiency in us, it is often because we are projecting an unrealistic ideal of perfection onto them. When that happens, we either have to change our outlook or change who we follow.

We have to keep bringing our attention back to the lives we already have, tethering ourselves to what is here and what is real: love, laughter, kind words, quiet beauty. The tiny details that make up the texture of our lives.

Seeing the beauty in imperfection

When a potter makes a series of handcrafted pots, they are not aiming for perfection in terms of symmetry and uniformity, or else they would use a machine. They aim for natural beauty, the mark of the hand, and the infusion of the heart.

We are not supposed to be flawless and uniform, as if we have come out of a people factory. What if you imagined yourself as a beautiful handcrafted pot, lovingly shaped and appreciated because of, not in spite of, your imperfections? What if you acknowledged that texture, character, and depth are what underlie your natural beauty, inside and out? And what if you recognized how all that has shaped you along the way has made you who you are today?

Over the years, we paste layers over our natural beauty in our endless pursuit of perfection—with antiaging creams, accumulated stuff, job titles, and projected images that we think might make other people like us better. But all that is heavy and it masks what lies within. It's only when you strip back the layers that you let your inner beauty shine.

It is our imperfections that make us unique, and our uniqueness that makes each of us beautiful.

What if we were to agree that our ideal state is actually perfect imperfection and that we are already there? There would be no more struggle or exhausting hustle. Rather, a relaxing into the knowledge that we are just fine, just as we are.

Going one step further, we might see that those imperfections could actually be the doorways to new learning opportunities, experiences, conversations, and connections. Suddenly, perfect would not seem so desirable after all, and we would realize that we are capable of more than we have ever imagined.

Let's cast our minds back to what the monk said in chapter 3. "*Wabi sabi* is naturalness, it's about things in their natural, most authentic state." What does your "natural, most authentic state" look like? Is that how you walk through the world? Is that the version you take with you to work? Or the version you show to your friends and family? If not, what do you need to strip away to get back to that state?

Letting go of perfect

Frank Ostaseski, founding director of the Zen Hospice Project in San Francisco, once said: "Wholeness does not mean perfection. It means no part left out."[2]

I am writing this at my kitchen counter, glass of wine in hand, dinner dishes stacked high in the sink, waiting for some attention. A voice in my head keeps reminding me that my large travel bag is still lying on my bedroom floor, in the exact spot I left it there on Sunday after my latest trip away. At my feet are strewn children's toys—an open jewelry box with a sleepy ballerina done with pirouetting for the day, a little teapot ready to serve a teddy bear's picnic, a balloon from a long-forgotten party slowly wrinkling up . . .

To begin with, I found so much about parenting not just challenging but also confusing. To at once feel so blessed yet so frustrated. So deeply grateful for their presence yet stressed out by their demands. So utterly in love yet out of control. And then I realized it's not just the children who are growing but us parents, too. We need space to grow into the parents we are becoming. The discomfort is growth. That's why it's scary, difficult, and chaotic, but look what it leads to.

Now I look around at the chaos on my living-room floor—the half-dressed doll and rabble of Duplo blocks, the pile of books and scattering of abandoned crayons—and I see something else. I see their incessant curiosity, boundless energy, and burning desire to learn more about the world around them. I see joy. Unadulterated child's play. There's medicine in their laughter and wonder in the air.

I have done my best to make our home soulfully simple and quietly beautiful. But I am not going to kid myself that I should be some kind of perfect homemaker or that my house is going to be tidy all the time.

I think about how I want my daughters to remember their childhood. Is the most important thing for them to say, "We always had a perfectly tidy house"? No. I'm not judging you if you do have a tidy house. I am secretly jealous of it. But what I am saying is that we have to make choices and right now this is mine. I want them to say, "Our house was a lovely happy house, where we felt safe and comfortable. We were always loved and looked after, and we were taught how to love and look after one another. We learned to treasure what we had, and even more than that, to treasure our time together."

"Don't worry. It won't last," people say. But that's also the sad thing, and the reason for seeking the gift among it all. Because it won't last. My girls will soon be interested in different things, different people. They won't want to snuggle in close, play for hours, or chatter with me all day long. And so now, while it lasts, I'm going to be grateful for all of it. Even the wrinkly balloon bobbing around my feet.

Accepting the hard stuff

Everything in nature is changing, and so is your story. Acceptance doesn't mean this is how it's going to end. It's an acknowledgment that this is where it begins. We are all works in progress. To be alive is to evolve. You can play an active role in that evolution, but first you need to recognize that it is happening. *Wabi sabi* helps you to do that in a gentle and nourishing way.

Wabi sabi teaches perspective—seeing things for how big or small they really are, whether they really matter, and whether to nourish them or let them go. When something hard is happening, acceptance can be a real friend. It's not about handing over your power, or allowing inappropriate behavior. It's not passive, it's active.

Acceptance means saying:

1. This is what is happening (observing it, not resisting it).
2. This is how much it really matters (if at all).

3. This is the beginning of all that is to come, and this is what
   I am going to do next.

It's saying: This is where I am. This is where we are. The vase
is smashed. The marriage is broken. The business is struggling. I
am lonely. My child is upset. I just got rejected again. Whatever
is going on, this is what is, right now. We mustn't ignore what's
happening, but we also don't need to dramatize it. We need to live
and acknowledge it, and then let go of the attachment to it. The
truth is, we can't hold on and we can't just push on past; when we
learn to surrender to difficulty, accepting that it will come and it
will go, life shifts from a battle to a dance.

Allowing the future

Not long ago I spent time in the home of Mineyo Kanie, a wonderful ninety-four-year-old woman you will meet in chapter 8.
When prompted for her secret to a happy life, she said she
believed the root of all unhappiness was not being content with
what you have and spending too much time looking outside
your life instead of spending time inside it. This doesn't mean
we cannot have dreams, but rather that happiness begins with
gratitude. Kanie-*san* has clearly seen the *tsukubai* at Ryōan-ji, too
(see page 90).

Hope is not the same as expectation. You can plan for and
invite a particular future, but you cannot determine or control
it. Visualize what you want, but then let it go. Release your
attachment to the timeline and then come back to being present
in your life right now.

This week, I challenge you to get clear on what you are grateful for and then let go of all expectation about anything that has

not yet happened. Open your mind and heart to whatever might unfold. Try to go a whole seven days without having to control everything, without stressing when things don't work out as you thought they would or should. As you do this, any time you feel the need to take charge, try to relax out of it, just to see what happens. Look for the good that happened precisely because things didn't work out the way you thought they would or should.

And take your time. There really is no desperate hurry. When we constantly pursue perfection, our life speeds up. We make hasty decisions and snap judgments. *Wabi sabi* offers an opportunity to pause, reflect, check in with yourself, and move on from there. You'll likely feel relieved and make better choices.

Stay open. Make room for small miracles.

WABI SABI–INSPIRED WISDOM FOR ACCEPTANCE + LETTING GO

- *Change is inevitable, so trying to hold on to the past or present is pointless. Be open. Your life is happening right here, right now.*
- *When your head cannot find the answers, remember your heart may know the way.*
- *Perfection is a myth. You are perfectly imperfect, just as you are.*

TRY IT: PRACTICING ACCEPTANCE

Acceptance is a decision (I am not going to be caught up in a whirlwind of thoughts pulling me away from being here), a recognition (this is what has just happened or what is happening right now), and a new beginning (by realizing where I am, I can move forward from here, with this as my new starting point).

Whatever is going on for you right now, consider trying to accept it in this moment, and see what difference it makes to your perspective. Use the exercise below to help you do this:

1. **The decision:** I am not going to get caught up in a whirlwind of thoughts, pulling me away. (Describe where you are, what you can see/hear/taste/smell/feel with your body, such as your feet on the floor or the feel of the seat you are sitting on.) Right now, in this moment I am:

   _____

   _____

   _____

2. **The recognition:** this is what has just happened or what is happening right now. The facts in this moment are:

   _____

   _____

   _____

3. **The new beginning:** this is a new beginning. (This doesn't have to be a dramatic new beginning, although it can be.) With this starting point I can/I will:

   _____

   _____

   _____

Acceptance isn't always easy. Things happen that feel unfair, uninvited, badly timed, painful. It's not a way to numb your emotions, but rather a way to get some clarity to allow you to feel what you need to feel. At a time like this, self-care is paramount. Make a commitment to yourself.

Ways in which I am going to take care of myself as I go through this:

❋ **Mind** (e.g., share my worries with a friend, say no to additional commitments this week):

_____

_____

_____

_____

_____

❋ **Body** (e.g., go for a long walk in nature, nourish my body with fresh and wholesome food):

_____

_____

_____

_____

_____

❋ **Spirit** (e.g., meditate first thing in the morning, keep a gratitude list):

_____

_____

_____

_____

_____

七転び八起き

CHAPTER 5:
REFRAMING
FAILURE

The Japanese have a famous proverb, 七転び八起き, *nana korobi, ya oki*, meaning, "Fall down seven times, get up eight." This is something I became intimately familiar with when learning Japanese. The proverb represents the idea of not giving up, but more than that, it doesn't start with falling down (as that would be "fall down seven times, get up seven.") It counts the first time you get up, reminding us that we have to show up first, in order to have the chance to fail, and then have the chance to get back up again.

As the only nonlinguist on my degree course, things don't begin well. In the first week of university, when my new friends are learning lofty things in labs and lecture theaters, I am practicing how to say "Hello" in three different ways, depending on the time of day. And sometimes getting it wrong.

As a student in the Department of East Asian Studies at Durham University, I love the tradition and the experience—the small group tutorials with kind teachers in classrooms tucked into the eaves of an old Victorian house, the rows and rows of books with kanji characters on their spines, which I dream of being able to read one day, and the Oriental Museum next door, packed with textiles, woodblock prints, and other exotic artifacts. Our lessons include learning the etiquette of visiting Japanese people's homes, watching Miyazaki animations, and spending Thursday afternoons dipping brushes into shiny black ink to paint kanji on rice paper, with classical music playing in the background.

Japanese is a song, and I love the sound of it. I am just not very good at singing it.

From the very first vocabulary test, my path is littered with the debris of failure. I do so badly in my first-year exams that one of the senior lecturers calls me into his office and announces, with a solemn look on his face, that the department isn't sure if they should let me go to Kyōto the following term. What? Don't they understand? Going to live in Japan has been the whole point. I am here for the adventure. I beg and plead and assure them that I will be fine once I spend time immersed in the language and culture. Somehow it works, and a few weeks later I find myself on a plane heading east, self-doubt tucked into my suitcase alongside my kanji dictionary and a year's worth of clothes.

Walking through Kansai International Airport, I see signs I can't read, hear conversations and announcements I can't understand, and I am floored by the realization that people actually speak the language of my textbooks. The same one I should have spent hours studying instead of broadcasting the news bulletin on the university radio or gathering campus gossip for the student paper. And then I meet my host mother, who only speaks Kyōto dialect, and the rest of my host family, none of whom speaks English, and it suddenly becomes very clear that I'll have to up my game if I am going to survive the next year.

My language-learning journey, drawn on a graph, starts at zero at the bottom left, with a nervous line indicating a rocky start, followed by a general lift the first year I am in Kyōto. The line rises in times of high motivation and dips in times of low morale. It plateaus about halfway through, rises again with approaching exams, and rises further on my return to England, as I finish my degree. I get to a point where I feel quite confident on graduation, only to get a shock on entering the workforce in Japan, seeing that the vertical axis reaches so much higher than I had realized. What I think of as a pretty good standard turns out not to be that good, after all, when I have to interpret live, on big stages, for governors, ambassadors, and top athletes. I tape meetings and relisten until I understand, painstakingly translate newspaper articles, and throw myself into as many cultural classes and friendships as I can. All the while, it is a roller coaster of pride and despair, as I alternate between how far I have come and how far I have to go.

Eventually, I come to realize that I can only do what I can do, with the tools I have in the moment. I can prepare myself as best as possible and then I just need to show up—ideally, well rested and alert—to do the best job possible. Every time I do this, I get a little better, learn a little more, and grow in confidence. Of course, there are times when that confidence is shattered all over again, but I pick myself up and get on with it.

That graph of language learning rose again with every year I spent working in Tōkyō. It probably peaked in the year I spent immersed in the study of simultaneous interpreting skills for my master's degree. It was then that I went to the UN for work experience, sharing an interpreting booth with women who were brought up bilingual, had three decades of experience in the job, and knitted as they switched effortlessly between languages. Going there was probably a mistake. I was hugely intimidated and felt my own confidence seeping away. My graph suddenly looked like the Nikkei index after a stock-market crash.

But this is what we do. The better we get at something, the more we widen our field of vision. We move from puddle to pond, from pond to sea. The ideal is always changing, and as long as we use that as the motivation to do more quality, heart-and-soul work, that's fine. But when it becomes an exercise in comparison, it's a dangerous place to be. I'm not saying you should settle for the puddle. I'm saying you might be happy in the pond, and that's okay if that's where you do your best. You might feel destined for the sea, and that's fine, too. Just be sure you go there for the right reasons.

How is this connected to *wabi sabi*? It is the relief that comes from knowing that nothing is ever permanent, perfect, or complete. When I mess up, it's a blip, not a life sentence. When I make a mistake, I can correct it or do things better next time.

There is no "done," "complete," or "perfect" with learning. There is just learning.

Wherever I am on my journey of learning, I am still traveling, not at the end of the line, which allows me to relax in the knowledge that I'm not supposed to know everything and makes me curious about what else there is to learn.

There is always the potential for a dip in the graph, for a plateau, or for a rise. It simply depends on you, your attitude, energy, and attention. This doesn't just go for learning a skill. It's true with learning about finances, or love, or parenting. Even about ourselves. There is no done, complete, or perfect. There is just learning.

The Japanese attitude to failure

In the course of my research, one of the major questions I had to grapple with was how to reconcile the *wabi sabi*–inspired notion of imperfection with the well-documented aversion to public failure in Japan. If a business fails, the CEO usually takes personal responsibility. The Asian economic crisis of the 1990s saw a domino toppling of some of the top figures in the country. And it's not just those in the public eye—every year, most students spend hours attending after-school *juku* (cram schools) to prepare for high school and university entrance exams in order to avoid missing out on a prized place. People in Japan don't like failure any more than anyone else, and there is still a social stigma attached to "losing face" when things don't work out.

What I have come to realize is that reframing failure does not mean learning to love it or welcoming it. It means doing your best with the intention of not failing (because you care about what you are doing), but if failure happens, then it means learning to deal with it in a way that helps you move forward.

In the *Disrupting Japan* podcast, an interview with Hiroshi Nagashima, founder of failed company Sharebu Kids, illustrates this brilliantly.[1] In his introduction, the host, Tim Romero, a veteran of start-ups in Japan, said: "Failure hurts. Failure is lonely. Some people who you thought were close friends stop returning your calls. Failure is where you see both the absolute worst and sometimes the absolute best in both yourself and the people around you."

When the company of Tim's guest, Mr. Nagashima, went south, his circle of investors, friends, and family were actually more accepting and supportive than he expected. The hardest part was how he initially beat himself up. However, in the end, Mr. Nagashima had a very clear view of what he would do differently if he did it again, and he managed to use his experience to land a good job in another company. He said the experience of failure, however difficult at the time, had strengthened him as a person, built his resolve, changed his perspective, and made him worry less about things that don't really matter.

In order to reframe failure, we first have to reframe success. When we set ourselves up with a singular goal and hang our personal worth on whether or not we achieve it—even if many of the contributing factors are beyond our control—the fall can be painful. This singular goal is caught up in our idea of perfection. "If only I achieve X, become Y, make Z . . . I will be happy."

Instead, if we change our view of success to one about how we want to feel and how we want to experience life, everything changes with that. We discuss this further in chapter 7, but for now, let's look at what we can learn about failure when we approach it with a *wabi sabi* worldview:

1. We don't have to like failure to learn from it. Failure builds our resilience and helps us grow in other ways. And when we stop trying to be perfect, we might not even see the "failure" as a "failure" anymore.

2. The feeling of failure won't last for ever. Nothing is permanent. Each day is an opportunity for a new beginning.

3. Everything is changing. Perhaps this is a moment to pause, pivot, and pursue something else.

The perils of pursuit

Competition is not a bad thing. It encourages us to challenge ourselves and hone our craft. The issue comes when we try to pursue perfection in a world where so much is beyond our control. Our risk of failure is a product of the size of the stage we put ourselves on. Anyone can win at anything if the stage is small enough. The growth opportunity is in the stretching, which will inevitably mean there are times when we don't win. But if we see it from the beginning for what it is—us expanding our comfort zone and opening our hearts to an even bigger experience—then it's a gift.

When we try our luck on a bigger stage and it doesn't work out, it's not a failure, it's a moment of expansion.

As an interpreter, I have stood side by side with numerous world-class athletes who have fallen short of their goals on the global stage, as well as with others who have won Olympic medals. I understand the emotional chasm between winning and losing. I have lived the depth of disappointment in the immediate aftermath of missing a goal for which so much has been sacrificed along the way. But without exception, those who go on to greater things are those who realize this: the important thing is what happens next.

It's the same with filmmaking, with cake baking, with academic achievement—indeed, in any arena where we chase a specific dream. We have a choice in any moment of perceived failure, about what we do with it and how we move forward.

Be ambitious. Be talented. Be amazing. Pursue inspiring dreams and delight in the steps along the way. But don't pursue that elusive ego-driven perfection. Instead, relax in the knowledge that perfection is an unattainable goal. It's the expansion that matters.

Practicing expansion

My Japan connection has led me to some unusual jobs over the years, perhaps none more so than as an interpreter for a long-distance swimmer who was attempting to traverse the English Channel in under fifteen hours. Ken Igarashi is a rice farmer from the coastal city of Tsuruoka. A keen swimmer in junior high school, he then fell into work and family life, leaving the swimming behind. In his twenties he took up weight lifting, and this strength would serve him well when he returned to long-distance swimming in his midthirties.

When I met him, a decade or so later, he was already the first Japanese person to have swum the Tsugaru Strait, the body of water between Honshū and Hokkaidō, which connects the Sea of Japan with the Pacific Ocean. He traveled to Dover with his coach, and the three of us stayed in a cozy B and B with seagulls calling outside. The rules for attempting a cross-Channel swim from England to France are strict, not least because of the dangers of crossing a major shipping lane. We had a set window for the swim, and an independent adjudicator would accompany the coach and me on a pilot boat alongside Ken. We were able to throw him drinks and food attached to a thin rope, but if the rope went taut the attempt was off. If he touched the boat at any time, the attempt was off. Regardless of whether he got a cramp, was stung by a jellyfish, or anything else along the way, we were not allowed to offer any physical assistance whatsoever to the Vaseline-covered man in a Speedo alongside our boat.

On the designated day of his swim, I woke around 3 a.m., had a cheese sandwich, and went to the lobby to meet Ken and his coach. To my dismay, Ken was groggy and swaying. It turned out that the sleeping pills and whiskey he had imbibed the night before to help get over the jet lag had not mixed well and, on any normal day, he would have been advised to go back to bed. I did not want him to step into the sea, in the dark, in that state, but he insisted he had only one window to try it. Ultimately, the decision rested with his coach and, after a careful assessment, he gave the green light.

Things did not begin well. The challenge starts the moment you step off the shore at Dover and into the water, so the clock was already ticking when bizarrely, just a few hundred feet out, Ken started swimming back to England. The adjudicator was understandably concerned at his disorientation. The coach shouted some instructions and encouraged him to face France again, and off we went.

The shock of the cold and the realization of the error seemed to shake him fully awake, and after that it was a solid show of perseverance for many hours. However, that initial mistake cost him dearly at the end. There is a point close to Calais that juts farther into the sea than any other part of the shoreline. If you are fast enough in reaching it, you can shave a significant amount off your final time. Unfortunately, Ken just missed it, and with the effect of the tide, he ended up swimming a further two hours.

As soon as he climbed back into the boat, shivering and exhausted but jubilant that he had reached France, he was interviewed by NHK, Japan's national broadcaster, via satellite phone. Asked about his challenge Ken replied, "*Isshōkenmei ganbarimashita.*" "I gave it my all."

By the harshest of standards, Ken had failed to reach his fifteen-hour goal, eventually finishing in sixteen hours and forty-two minutes. However, he had still swum the Channel—a monumental effort—so he focused on what he had achieved and was proud that he had tried his best and pushed himself to complete his first international crossing. There is also no doubt he took away some major learning for his future challenges.

That attitude took him far. Ken Igarashi, whose family name means "Fifty Storms," went on to become the first Japanese person to swim from Japan to Korea, from Japan to Russia, and all the way across Lake Baikal.

TEN WAYS TO NURTURE RESILIENCE

1. Boost your physical vitality, with exercise, nourishment, and rest.
2. Boost your mental vitality with quiet time, adequate sleep, and time in nature.
3. Practice coping with small things so you can better cope with the big things.
4. Set yourself a series of small goals and work toward them.
5. Grow something. Pay attention to the difference your care makes.

6. Make regular notes of the things you do well, to remind you how capable you are.
7. Seek out community and build a support network.
8. Seek out resilience role models and learn from them.
9. Surround yourself with inspiring quotes.
10. Look for reasons to be positive every day.

But it's hard . . .

. . . I know it's hard. The kind of failure that turns to regret and self-bashing is heavy. The job you didn't get. Ouch. The years you spent in a relationship with someone who crushed your spirit. Ouch. The fifteenth publisher that rejected your book proposal. Ouch. The project you agreed to without a contract, which then went south. Ouch. The time you said yes, when you knew in your gut it should have been a no. Ouch all over again.

No one's saying it's easy to fail. But the good news is, you get to choose what you do with it. If you try to hold the failure in that place of regret and self-bashing, it will only morph into something darker and heavier. Because everything changes, right? Instead, try to encourage it to transform into a lesson. However hard this may seem, you have the power to make that choice at any time. Focus on what would be different if you excavated the teaching instead.

Resistance to the possibility of failure

In my work helping people transition between careers, between lifestyles, and between life stages, I constantly come across resistance to being a beginner, due to an overwhelming fear of failure.

If you start something new, it's highly likely you will get things wrong along the way.

There's no doubt this is hard on the spirit as well as on the ego. It's easy to see why so many people spend years on a track that is making them miserable now, to avoid the possibility of a mistake making them miserable in the future. This is particularly the case with people wanting to shift into a more creative way of living or earning their income from a creative profession. The risk is too high, the fear of failure too great, the ghosts of art teachers and other critics from the past too loud in their ears. But there is something they don't realize: failing your way forward is progress. Each time you do it, you build up your store of inner wisdom, to draw on next time you need it. The "failure" does not have to be the end of the story. It can be the beginning of the next chapter, but only if you accept the imperfection, show yourself compassion, and choose to move forward.

We have to stop telling ourselves that everyone is watching, waiting for us to fail. They really aren't.

No one is watching . . .

Cross-legged on a small cushion in a temple in Kyōto, I'm getting it all wrong. I'm supposed to be meditating, but all I can think of is the pins and needles in my legs, the shuffling noise as I try to get more comfortable, the voices in my head telling me everyone must be looking at me disapprovingly for being such a distraction. I can't resist sneaking a look around. Of course, no one is looking at me. No one cares what I am doing or whether I am doing it "properly." They are too busy doing their own thing.

Over here it's just me, judging myself, telling myself I've failed before I've actually thought through what "success" even means in a meditation. Only when I let go of the judgment do I finally relax into the moment and the setting, the faint sound of a bell, the discomfort as my ankles push against the floor, the smell of fresh tatami, the swish of the gardener raking the garden outside, the remembering that I am on an adventure and I chose to be here today.

SIX STRESS-FREE STEPS TO LEARNING FROM FAILURE

Use the six steps below to process any particular event or situation that you are hanging on to as a "failure":

1. **Truth** State the facts about what happened.
2. **Humility** Get clear on who you have been blaming and what role you played.
3. **Simplicity** Excavate your single greatest learning from the situation.
4. **Impermanence** Identify what was lost, what was gained, and what has changed inside you.
5. **Imperfection** Acknowledge what imperfection—in yourself or in someone else—you must forgive or embrace to move on, and remind yourself that imperfection makes you human.
6. **Incompleteness** Recognize that this is not the end of the story. Decide what you will do next.

Overcoming the fear of creative failure

We do our best creative work when we are at our most open and honest. That's when the results of our creativity connect deeply with others, expressing things we might never say in conversation. But sharing that which comes from deep inside can make us feel vulnerable, exposed, afraid: What if it's criticized, ridiculed, or rejected? That would feel like *we* are being criticized, ridiculed, or rejected. So it's no surprise that in my work supporting people to build a creative career, this comes up time and again.

The fear of failure is one of the most significant barriers to people doing what they love. And herein lies one of *wabi sabi*'s most important lessons. *Wabi sabi* is an intuitive response to beauty that reflects the true nature of life. It can be a response in someone else to the beauty of your creativity, which has come from within you. This means your creativity has to be shared in order for its beauty to be truly seen.

So for all of us who are hiding our creative expression for fear of failure, we are missing the point. The true beauty is not in the achievement of some kind of perfection but rather in the sharing of the creation itself.

Of course, there are many measures of "success" these days, depending on which metrics you favor. Did you sell out your art show? Did your book make the bestseller list? Did you have hundreds of Instagram followers liking your most recent post? These things matter insofar as they can help you make a living, which lets you do your creative thing more of the time, and we will explore this further in chapter 7. But these metrics do not matter at all in terms of the beauty you and the observers of your work are creating together. The only failure there would be in avoiding creating in the first place.

Giving it a try

It's not easy to deal with a fear of failure with something as personal as creativity, but try reframing that fear as an indicator of what you really care about and go for it anyway.

It is a balmy spring morning and I find myself strolling through the Nishijin textile district, home of weaving in Kyōto for more than fifteen hundred years and a stone's throw from the apartment my now-husband Mr. K and I have rented for six months. Nishijin is a fascinating area of the city, where you can see artisans at work, not for the benefit of tourists, but because they are simply doing their jobs, as many generations of talented people have done before them. One particular building catches my eye. It is a large wooden warehouse with a wide, welcoming entranceway, in front of which hangs a traditional noren curtain, announcing that the shop is open for business. Intrigued, I find myself peeking inside.

On stepping through the heavy sliding door, I gasp. It is a 3,200-square-foot workshop, with a triple-height vaulted ceiling. Flanked on both sides with some of the most beautiful kimonos I have ever seen, the central space is empty but for a couple of low tables, some sketching paper, and a pot of pens.

The building turns out to be the workshop of Kyōji Miura, an award-winning designer of high-end contemporary kimonos for geisha and couture customers. He also has a line in noren curtains, like the one that signaled me inside, and suddenly I really want to know how to make one.

I call a polite greeting into the vast space, and a kindly looking man with a long silver ponytail strolls out of a small room in the back corner. I am sorry for the interruption but wonder would it be possible to take a closer look at his beautiful work? A little bemused by this random foreigner who has wandered in off the street, he nods and indicates for me to go ahead.

After we have shared a cup of green tea and I have asked him a barrage of questions about his kimono designing, I sum up the courage to ask if he would teach me how to make a noren.

"Erm, I don't teach," he says awkwardly. "I just design."

"Ah, I see," I say, and wait.

"But then I suppose I could consider it. Why don't you come back tomorrow with a sketch of what you would like to make and I'll think about it."

I race home and eagerly make a mock-up, using washi *paper and a chopstick. He seems surprised when I return the following day, and even more so when I fish out the design from my backpack.*

"Hmm. Interesting. Not bad," he says, looking from the mock-up to me and back again.

And with that my apprenticeship begins. I spend many days in his studio, as things are sketched out and masked out, dyed and dried, stretched and washed.

There are many times during the process when I feel overwhelmed with the enormity of what I am trying to learn in a relatively short space of time. He is a master with incredibly high standards; I am a novice with no idea. But Miura-sensei continuously reminds me to focus on the task at hand. To keep on showing up at his studio, trying and seeing what happens. He teaches me to pay attention to the details and listen to the instructions, but also to use my instinct. After all, it is my design. In the mind of this particular master, there are no mistakes, just interesting creative experiments.

Back in Miura-sensei's studio, when we finally cut the long piece of hand-dyed linen into three panels, stitch them together, and hang them over a bamboo rail, I think my heart will burst. There are some uneven patches of dye, a wobbly line here and there, and a slight mismatch in the lining up of the panels. But to me, my first ever noren *is perfectly imperfect and something to be treasured.*

The curtain, which now hangs in my home, shows a silvery moon on an indigo background with two birds silhouetted against it. The pair of birds represent possibility, support, and freedom. And isn't that what we make space for when we overcome the fear of creative failure?

FIVE WAYS TO BUILD CREATIVE CONFIDENCE

Use these top tips for building creative confidence so that you keep on putting your work out into the world. When you do that, there is nothing to fail.

1. Forget about the label (artist, writer, etc.) and just get busy creating.
2. Give your attention to the process, not the end product.
3. If something's not working, try something else (a new medium, material, teacher, angle).
4. Only half the responsibility is yours. Show up with an open heart and watch the universe step in to help.
5. Don't go it alone. Find a community of others who love what you love and support one another.

Lessons from the House of Light

Traveling through Japan's back country, it has taken me five hours, six trains, a bento lunch, and a box of Pocky to get to Tōkamachi, deep in the snow country of Niigata. A friendly taxi driver picks me up from the station, and I give him all my attention as I can see nothing beyond the ten-foot-high walls of snow on either side of the road. In between local history snippets and recommendations of nearby hot springs, he shares how the local community has been experimenting with a new breed of rice. I am so caught up in the difference in flavor profiles of Japan's most popular koshihikari *and the newer* shinnosuke *brands, both products of the neighboring paddy fields, that I hardly notice that we have arrived at our destination. When we pull up in front of the imposing Hikari no Yakata (the House of Light),[2] it takes my breath away.*

Floating on a snow cloud, a wide wooden staircase leads up to an imposing entranceway, flanked on either side by a wraparound pillared veranda some nine feet or so above the ground. Designed for the Echigo-Tsumari Art Triennale as a habitable installation and a place for meditation by Japanese architect Daigo Ishii and American light artist James Turrell, the House of Light is a study in the hidden dimensions of light as experience.

The house is constructed in an elegant sukiya[3] *style, with gently sloping gabled and hipped roofs.[4] Inside, the tatami-matted rooms have* yukimi shōji, *paper screens that can be raised like a sash window to allow viewing of the snow from the cozy retreat of your futon. At first, the building looks traditional, but on closer inspection, subtle design features make it an interactive art experience—from the fiber optics in the bath to the gentle internal lighting intended to replicate the candlelight used in Japanese homes long ago.*

The House of Light can accommodate six people, but to my delight, the friendly manager greets me with the news that all the other guests have canceled, so I have the place to myself. What a precious gift this turns out to be.

Toward the end of the afternoon a local chef delivers a freshly cooked meal, consisting of ten different plates. As he explains each element in turn, I can't help thinking it's almost too indulgent for me, dining alone.

The room I choose to eat and sleep in is like no other. A huge square hole has been cut out of the white ceiling. At the touch of a button, the entire roof slides back to reveal the sky.

Just before sunset, a light show begins. The area surrounding the hole in the ceiling fades slowly from one color into another. Out of the window I can see snow and mountains and a gray-blue twilight; but above me, the pink light framing the hole has rendered the sky cerulean.

Chopsticks in hand, I do a silent bow to no one in particular. First for tasting is the simmered niimono, *a bowl of bamboo shoots, taro root,*

*enoki mushrooms, and sea bass. Then, as the sky turns green against its
pale cherry light frame, it's butterbur buds in sweet miso and sticky teriyaki
amberjack with ginger.*

*Now a pale indigo light takes over the ceiling and the sky looks yellow,
mirroring my rolled omelette, served with fern fronds and salmon. The sole
soup is next, beneath a sky that has brightened to azure against a cotton-
candy light frame. And now fried tōfu with carrot, as the pink brightens
and the sky shifts to a Persian blue.*

*The sky itself is only subtly changing as night falls, but the contrast
with the changing frame is extraordinary. White light makes for an
aubergine sky, mirroring the whiting and eggplant tempura on my plate.
Accompanying the rice and pale miso soup is a new shade of pink light,
which births a bright green sky. And then, as the meal is rounded off
with a smooth milk pudding, a bolt of sweet orange renders the sky a
jewel-tone turquoise.*

*Toward the end of the light show, appetite satiated, I clear the table
and settle into my futon on the tatami floor. The ceiling light drifts back
to an innocent white, rendering the sky indigo. The moon has been there
all the while. The night is clinging to the edges of the hole in the ceiling.
Just then, as I stare up at the infinite sky from the depths of my futon,
body warm but night air cold on my face, it starts to snow. Inside the room.*

*Real snow falling inside a real room. Outside in. Inside out. I know
I should close the roof, but I cannot move for thinking how this is not
supposed to happen, but how art has made it happen. How we perceive
and believe things have to be a certain way until we realize that that isn't
true. How anything is possible with the right conditions. And it makes me
wonder: How else are we limiting ourselves? What else could be possible
if we stopped telling ourselves the opposite?*

*Each time the border transitions from one color to another, the square
piece of sky inside it is also transformed. When we get stuck, it's as if we
are only seeing one version of the sky. We forget we are capable of seeing*

many different versions if only we change the frame. When we fail, it's not to say we should deny or run away from it, but rather recognize that we can transform our view of what has happened. Are we framing it with dark, heavy stories of regret and judgment? Shame and embarrassment? Disappointment and despair? Or are we framing it more lightly, as an opportunity to learn and grow, with courage and clarity, as a clue to possibly rethinking or changing direction? Or simply as a gentle reminder that we are human and people make mistakes? Shrinking or growing? Blame or possibility? Regret or learning opportunity? What we see changes depending on how we frame it. And that changes everything.

I am lost in these thoughts when suddenly everything goes black. The frame of light has disappeared. I suddenly feel sucked into the wide-open sky, almost as if I am falling upward toward it, and then the night wraps its cloak around me.

The next morning I wake to silence. Feet of snow are stacked up around the house and there is not a soul in sight. I had fallen asleep looking out over the village below, lights twinkling in the night, but then a mist moved in and now I cannot see beyond the trees. It's one hundred shades of white and gray outside.

I make myself cheese on toast in the fish grill and tea in a see-through pot. Then I just sit a little longer. I know there is something waiting for me in the space between what I saw and what I understood. I want to know it, so I listen. And while I'm waiting, I remember that I took photos of the sky through the hole in the ceiling on both my digital camera and my iPhone. I wonder how they turned out, so I take a look. The results are astonishing.

With my DSLR, the sky is almost the same color in each picture, just slowly darkening with each image as it naturally would with the descending darkness. But the iPhone pictures are different, the sky varying in color with each change of frame, in much the same way my brain presented it to me.

The same sky looks different through different lenses. And with this the House of Light reveals its final lesson to me: Our perception of our problems depends not just on how we frame them but also the lens through which we view them. We can look through a lens of judgment or a lens of grace, and that determines how much of an emotional toll we allow the "failure" to take.

The *sabi* beauty we spoke of in chapter 1 is not one that can be created by the human hand. In the same way, the lessons we learn from failure are not lessons we willingly create. Failure happens and there are different ways to deal with it, none of which involve you judging yourself for being a failure. How you experience and learn from failure all depends on the frame and the lens you choose.

Perhaps it's no coincidence that I learned this inside a structure built as a collaboration between a Japanese architect and a Western artist. Looking to other cultures, then back at our own, can be valuable. Realizing that there is more than one way to see the world gives us options:

- Framing and reframing.
- Grace not guilt.
- Falling up. Not falling down.

 WABI SABI—INSPIRED WISDOM
FOR REFRAMING FAILURE

- *There is no "complete" or "perfect" with learning. There is just learning.*
- *Failure is simply a moment of expansion. Failing your way forward is progress.*
- *Reframing failure transforms our experience of it.*

TRY IT: REFRAMING

Think of an example where you failed at something. In combination with the Six Stress-free Steps to Learning From Failure
on page 118, make some notes in response to the following
questions:

❀ What happened?

❀ What made you consider it a failure?

❀ How did you feel about it when it happened?

❀ Were you sufficiently prepared at the time?

❀ What were the external factors at play?

❀ Did you listen to your intuition? What was it telling you?

❀ Faced with the same situation in the future, what would
   you do differently?

❀ How can you reevaluate this failure with a growth reframe
   or through a lens of grace?

❀ What has changed as a result of the experience?

❀ What do you need to do now to move on from it?

Reflect on your answers and make notes beginning with:
"Thanks to [insert details of the event], I now . . . "

人との絆

CHAPTER 6:
NURTURING
RELATIONSHIPS

Hamana-sensei *has set delicate peach blossoms and a sprig of yellow rapeseed flowers in a bamboo vase, set off to one side of the* tokonoma *alcove. A hanging scroll bears the calligraphy* "Everyday heart," *scribed by a monk from Myōshin-ji Temple. I sit in the* seiza *position, legs folded beneath me, on a low, flat cushion on the tatami floor, beside my friend Izumi, who has been studying tea with Hamana-sensei for years.*

Resplendent in a black kimono, Hamana-sensei shuffles gracefully in and out of the tearoom, bringing tea utensils and a tiny lacquered pot of vibrant green matcha *tea powder. A* tsurigama *(hanging iron kettle) swings gently over charcoal in the* ro *(the sunken fire pit, set in the floor), as if a breeze is blowing through the room. Winter is leaving and spring is on its way.*

We sit in silence, watching, listening, savoring. Hamana-sensei is a gentle and welcoming host, his movements communicating all he needs to say as he prepares the tea for us. Mine is served in a raku-style tea bowl, deep black with a subtle luster, vertical sides shaped skillfully by hand. When I curl my fingers around the bowl, it feels like an extension of my own hands. Izumi's bowl is shallower with sloping sides, the color of pale earth. The tea is a bewitching forest green, with a delicate froth. Paired with seasonal blossom-shaped sweets, its bitter taste is refreshing.

Charcoal glows in the ro.
Early spring rain drumming.
No hurry today.

Japanese aesthetics are embodied in the traditional tea ceremony without being explicitly taught. Hamana-sensei almost never speaks of philosophy in his classes, yet I leave with the sense that I have learned something significant. It is just the ritualized making of tea, and yet it is so much more. The three of us have given and received, and been present for one another.

Lessons from the tearoom

In the olden days, samurai would remove their swords and hang them on the *katana-kake* (sword rack) before entering a tearoom through the *nijiri-guchi* (crawling-in entrance)—a door so small that everyone, regardless of status, would have to stoop and crawl through it. The tearoom compresses the world to that space, the present moment, the shared experience. Inside, everyone is equal. The host and guests offer one another care and consideration. They are mindful and accommodating of one another. They are grateful for what is being shared.

The foundation of the tea ceremony is a set of four principles known as *wa kei sei jaku* (和敬清寂): harmony, respect, purity, and tranquility.[1]

Wa (harmony)

This is the ideal nature of the interaction between the host and the guests, and the interplay between the season, utensils used, food served, and prevailing mood at a tea gathering. By extension, it can be considered the ideal nature of the interaction between people in everyday life. It is a feeling of oneness with nature and others, and a sensitivity to each other. Harmony leads to comfortable, drama-free relationships that can bring us a sense of peace.

Kei (respect)

This comes from accepting other people, as they are, where they are. It's also something we receive when we offer kindness and humility. Both the host and the guests treat the tea utensils with care and respect, and the guests gratefully appreciate the setting and details, which the host has prepared with them in mind. The host and guests are considerate of and present with one another, as we can be in daily life.

Sei (purity)

Purity refers both to the importance of cleanliness and the attention to detail in the tea ceremony. Traditionally, guests at a tea gathering pass along a *roji* (garden path) and wash their hands and mouth at a small stone basin before entering the tearoom. As they walk the path, guests transition from the noisy, dirty world of everyday life into the pure, quiet space of the tearoom. *Sei* also refers to a purity of heart and freedom from attachment to things and status, reminding us to seek out the best in one another in a trusting, caring, nonjudgmental way.

Jaku (tranquility)

Jaku is an active state of stillness—a feeling of serenity. According to the Urasenke school of tea, although a person can work toward attaining each of the first three principles (harmony, respect, and purity) in turn, this last is attained through the constant practice of the other three. Urasenke says "a person whose heart inclines towards Tea is prepared to approach the utter stillness and silence of jaku."[2] Remaining calm, whatever is going on in our lives, allows us to think clearly and respond appropriately.

These four principles have been handed down over the centuries to provide guidance in the tearoom and can bring serenity to our everyday lives. To this day, they offer a gentle framework for approaching our relationships with others, both in everyday considerations and in times of particular conflict.

Think about how different each of your relationships—loving and challenging—could be with a little more attention to harmony, respect, purity, and tranquility.

Going easy on those we love

Mr. K has a habit of leaving wet tea towels on the side in our kitchen. It used to drive me nuts. Why can't he just hang the tea towel up on the rack? I'd ask myself as I replaced it over and over, sowing another tiny seed of frustration each time. I mentioned it a couple of times, and for a while he'd hang it up and then he'd forget and it would appear on the side again. I'd mull it over in my mind, usually when I should be doing something else: I wonder if other people's husbands do this, too? Am I the only one who has to tidy up after my other half, as well as my children? (Which, by the way, is totally unfair to Mr. K, who is tidier than me.)

And then one day it hit me. The only reason the tea towel was on the side was because he had just washed up, dried up, and put everything away. And that was after he had made the dinner, told a story to our girls, given me a hug, and asked me about my day. It was after he had made us all laugh, dancing around the kitchen, and shared a secret over a cup of tea. I have so much appreciation for Mr. K, and yet—somehow—I had become fixated on the wet tea towel on the side. In the end, I just let it go. And now, each time I pick up that wet tea towel and hang it on the rack, I choose to see it as a symbol of all I am grateful for in him.

Just as we are not perfect, neither is anyone else. What difference would it make if you saw others with your heart instead of seeing and judging with your eyes and mind? If you let go of the judgment and frustration and accepted who they are without trying to change them? If you don't like what you find, that's useful information and you can choose what to do next. But just maybe that acceptance will give you perspective and remind you of what really matters.

A *wabi sabi*–inspired worldview opens up a space for love.

Generosity of spirit: look for the good

Wanting to understand how all this connects back to Zen and *wabi sabi*, I sat down with Reverend Takafumi Kawakami, deputy head priest of Shunkō-in Temple in Kyōto. He explained the Buddhist concept of *kū*, which is often translated as "emptiness" or "no self." According to Reverend Kawakami, this idea is less about the absence of a self and more about a sense of oneness with everything.[3]

We are all interconnected and interdependent. We cannot exist without one another or without the world around us. This is why the connection we feel in the tea-ceremony room is so powerful. It's a moment to ponder and appreciate our relationship to one another. We are all busy living our own lives, but in that moment when we pause to enjoy the multisensory experience of the tea ceremony, we cross in time and space. We are reminded how the principles of *wa kei sei jaku* can bring compassion and calm to our deeply connected but sometimes frenetic lives.

Recently, I shared a lunch of *yuzu* rice and winter vegetables with my friend Ai Matsuyama, who I met many years ago when we were both training at the NTV College for TV Presenting. Our teacher was a veteran of Japanese television. The first time I opened my mouth to speak in class, she tilted her head in a concerned way and said, "Oh dear. You sound like a country bumpkin." (I had just moved to Tōkyō from a remote place in the north of Japan where the local accent was strong.) She gave me absolutely no consideration for the fact that when I was trying to read the news or do the weather or interview for vox pops in the street, I was doing it in a foreign language. She treated me exactly the same as all the Japanese students. And I loved her for it.

There were plenty of reasons for me to be nervous and feel under pressure in that class, but Ai always made me laugh out loud in class and never let me take myself too seriously. When we met up again this time, we went to a posh café and she made me laugh out loud inappropriately all over again. Ai is someone who lives on the bright side and always brings a wonderful energy to any gathering. I asked her to share the secret to her positivity. She said, "I always try to find at least one good thing in everyone, even people I don't really like." This generosity of spirit is an anonymous gift to the recipient, while making Ai's own experience of the relationship more pleasant. It's probably no coincidence that the character for Ai's name (愛) means "love."

Cultivating a generosity of spirit can transform our experience of relationships.

This sent me back to my conversation with Reverend Kawakami, during which he had suggested that humans tend to have confirmation bias: once we have decided someone is a "bad person" or a "good person," he said, we start looking for evidence to support our assumption, based on that existing bias. So the mind adds to the assumptions we have already made about someone. However, if we can recognize this and instead try to find evidence that we are wrong, it can make a huge difference in our relationships. This doesn't mean accepting inappropriate behavior or allowing people to bully or control us, but simply trying to see the good in people, even if we don't agree with them in every way.

If someone annoys you with a particular habit, you can do one of four things:

1. Say to yourself, "Here they go again" and add misery to the frustration.
2. If it is unbearable, take action to change your situation.
3. Accept their habit and give it no more attention.
4. Find something good in their habit, even if this is counter-intuitive.

It's up to you.

Helping others belong

One day, soon after I went to Kyōto to study, I was exploring a small back street behind the famous Philosopher's Path and I stumbled across a lovely little temple called Anraku-ji. It was closed, but its tiny side door was open a crack. Being a curious teenager, I pushed on it and peered inside. There, I found a lady called Mrs. Tanaka teaching basket weaving to a group of laughing Japanese women. She beckoned me over and invited me to join in.

It turned out Mrs. Tanaka's real talent was as an ikebana teacher and, thanks to her kindness, I ended up spending every Monday of the next year at her house after school, learning how to arrange and subtract flowers in the *Sōgetsu* style. There was no pressure or competition, just a safe place for connection and friendship. I was a lonely teenager in a foreign land. When she invited me through that gate, Mrs. Tanaka invited me into a world of beauty and culture and, more important, into her community.

This memory came flooding back when I was reading a recent study by Manchester Metropolitan University showing how the pressure to succeed is increasing the sense of loneliness among young people, with as many as one in three young people in the UK suffering from loneliness. The research cited "fear of failure and disappointing others, pressure from social media, major life changes, poverty and feeling different" as some of the issues that are having this impact.[4]

Although the study focused on young people, we can see this throughout society, regardless of age. All through education we are pitted against one another—academic results, sports days, music competitions, and so on, not to mention the popularity contest on social media. At work it's the same: Who got the promotion? Who won Employee of the Year? Who made the most sales? And in parenting, too: Whose child started to walk first? Spoke first? Won this trophy or passed that entrance exam? I'm not saying that we shouldn't be proud of our achievements and those of our nearest and dearest. Of course we should. But let's also be mindful of all that we celebrate—who we are, not just what we achieve, giving credit to the effort, as well as the wins.

The more we can show those we love that we honor and accept them in all their glorious imperfection, the more we can let them know they won't be judged or rejected if things don't always work out right. The more we can help them anchor themselves in what is real—not what they see on their phones—the more chance we have of helping them feel they belong.

Lessons from the jazz café

One August evening twenty-one years ago, I was with my band Blue Moon doing a gig in a dimly lit jazz café. I was on bass, my wife, Kyōko, was doing a moody vocal, and our friend Shibue-*san* was on drums. The door opened and in walked a young Englishwoman with a shock of peroxide-blond hair, a small backpack, and a big smile.

She waved at Shibue-*san* and then went to the bar and ordered a beer. When our set was over, Kyōko went over to talk to the woman, who had apparently just started working at Shibue-*san*'s office. (He was a government official by day and a drummer by night.) Within a couple of minutes, they were chatting animatedly. A few minutes later, the woman looked surprised and delighted. She started nodding her head and bowing.

I went over to see what was going on. "This is Beth," Kyōko said. "She just moved here from England. She doesn't have anywhere to stay, so I said she can come and live with us. You don't mind, do you?"

And so began the year when our home became known as the Adachi Hospital for Homesick Foreigners. We have a small music studio with a built-in bar and a grand piano in our slightly unusual house. During the time Beth lived with us, it was often filled with foreigners and Japanese people alike, who would come for parties, to listen to our jam sessions, and to learn how to make cocktails from our friend Fuji.

We'd often talk late into the night, sharing stories and hot stew as the snow fell outside. I spent many years abroad in my twenties and was the recipient of much kindness from the people I met along the way. I lived in London's Notting Hill way before it became a desirable place to be, doing odd jobs to buy food and fuel for my motorbike.

Having Beth in the house reminded me of my traveling days. She was full of energy and curiosity, always coming home from her job at the local government with funny stories about various people she had met or situations she had encountered.

These days, a lot has changed in all our lives, but we still share a common love of the simple things. Good conversation, cold beer, real friendship. I count my blessings every day, and the older I get, the more I value the gifts of a simple life.

This is how Michiyuki Adachi remembers the day we met. Adachi-*san* is one of the kindest, most generous, and most contented people I know. I think it's no coincidence that he is all those things at once. Now the president of a successful company, Adachi-*san* takes his entire workforce on overseas trips every couple of years, encourages laughter in the workplace, and has a staff turnover close to zero. It makes me smile to know that his name, Michiyuki, literally means "road-happiness" or as he might say, "enjoying the journey." He and his wife, Kyōko, taught me so much about how to find contentment. It starts with nurturing relationships with other people and ends with being grateful for it all.

Of course, there are times when we need to be cautious around strangers. But we have an in-built system of intuition to help us discern this, to keep ourselves safe. More often than not, the way you are treated as a traveler is a reflection of the way you travel. If you explore with an open heart and mind, that's usually how you are received, and this has always been my experience in Japan.

Face-to-face

In the course of my research for this book, almost everyone who generously agreed to be interviewed asked that I speak to them in person. In this age of free video chats, it can seem extreme to fly halfway around the world for a conversation, but it matters. The same sense of intuition that leads Japanese people to feel *wabi sabi* in the presence of beauty, guides them to read you as a person. They recognize how much lives between the words, in the unsaid, and there is nothing like a face-to-face for a heart-to-heart.

There is a phrase in Japanese, 空気を読む, *kūki o yomu*, which literally means "to read the air." It refers to the ability to sense an atmosphere, and act accordingly. The clues might come from body language, facial expressions, or simply a feeling. Being able to read the air facilitates harmony among a group, because it allows you to anticipate the needs of others without them specifically saying what they need, understanding when to speak and when to listen. This is not simply a Japanese trait. Anyone can do it with a combination of intuition, emotional intelligence, and empathy. It can be a valuable tool when trying to broach a tricky subject, share news that may not be well received, or simply show that you are in tune with someone else. Instead of simply seeing with your eyes and hearing with your ears, try experiencing a person and a conversation from your heart, by showing up fully and really listening. See what a difference it makes.

Calm rules

Japan consistently appears in the top ten most peaceful countries in the world, according to the Global Peace Index.[5] Danielle Demetriou of the *Telegraph* recently observed: "Tōkyō may be

one of the world's most densely populated cities but it is also a
city in possession of a calm and efficient rhythm that belies its
sprawling dimensions." She went on to note that "Kyōto moves
to an altogether different rhythm with its riverside cherry trees
bursting into cloudlike bloom and Zen gardens with raked sand
and *haiku*-inspiring rock formations."[6]

Beyond the packed subway trains, noisy *pachinko* parlors,[7] and
loud public announcements, there is an underlying calm that
invites you to relax and breathe deeply. Some might say this

A *wabi sabi*–
inspired world-
view can help
us invite calm
in the midst
of chaos.

has to do with the prevalence of temples and
shrines (there are more than two thousand
in Kyōto alone) and the pockets of nature
found everywhere. Others might say it is in
the Japanese aesthetic sense, which leads the
country to offer moments of stillness, simplicity, and beauty in the most unexpected
of places. Yet others would say it is to do
with the way people behave and interact with
one another.

Being able to access a place of calm in the midst of our tumul-
tuous lives can help us to cope, make better decisions, stay serene,
and communicate better with one another. It is good for mind and
body, because it helps us avoid flooding our systems with stress hor-
mones every time something unexpected or challenging happens.

There is a time and a place for excitement, euphoria, exhila-
rated joy, and even nervous anticipation. These kinds of extreme
emotions rarely exist alongside calm in the moment and are part
of diving deep into the experience of our lives. But living at the
extremes of emotion—whether up or down—for an extended
period of time is exhausting. Layering extreme emotions over
daily stress and uncertainty can cause chaos. Calm can be a

welcome tonic to bring us back into balance, offering clarity, serenity, and quiet genius.

It reminds us that everything is impermanent, imperfect, and incomplete, anyway, and encourages us to seek simplicity and serenity wherever we can.

Calm communication

At the turn of the millennium I found myself in Tōkyō, working on the organization of the 2002 FIFA World Cup Korea/Japan. Cohosting one of the world's biggest sporting events inevitably brought all sorts of operational and political challenges and delicate negotiations. Despite this, it was a rare meeting between the Japanese officials and their European and American counterparts where a voice was raised on the Japanese side.

One thing I learned during that time was the value of calm communication. There were vast differences of opinion, seemingly insurmountable problems, and real frustrations from all parties, not to mention the added layer of cross-cultural misunderstanding. Yet none of the issues was resolved with anger or verbal demonstrations of strength. With the help of skilled interpreters, the gentle way won the day.

We all want to be heard and understood, and keeping calm when we communicate can help us do that so much better. When someone talks to us in an aggressive way, forces an opinion on us, says something hurtful or something we strongly disagree with, we have a choice: we can choose to react in a way that escalates the negative energy and aggression, or we can choose to respond calmly in a way that brings a more considered discussion or even closure of the conversation. This isn't about always agreeing, or giving in, but it's about using calm tools to have better conversations and avoid additional stress.

More than words

We all communicate with our body language and facial expressions, with the tone of our voice and with our energy. Depending on what we choose to do with each of them, we can bring about an opening up or a shutting down. Once someone shuts down, it's hard for them to hear what you are trying to say, and if you allow yourself to get caught up in spiraling negative energy, it's also hard for you to hear someone else.

One of the most important things I learned about calm communication in Japan is this: you can communicate what you feel without reenacting how you feel. So if someone makes you feel angry, you can explain your point without shouting it. You can let someone know you are feeling stressed without snapping at them. And if you can do that, it's going to go better for everyone.

Within the context of people speaking Japanese, there is so much more that goes on beyond what is actually said. From the level of politeness and the depth of the bowing, to the atmosphere and shared understanding that somehow needs no words, there is infinitely more to Japanese than the words themselves. While it is hard to translate the subtleties of this, there are valuable things we can all take away: sensitivity, patience, real listening, consideration for others.

Lessons from the hot spring

I can remember clearly the precise moment I made the mistake.

It is one of those days when I am trying to power through a long list, I have a head cold, my eldest daughter is hanging off my arm as I try to type, and my youngest is scrabbling around my feet in search of a lost doll's shoe. I really should wait for a quiet moment to complete the booking, but I am running out of time before my trip, so I just go ahead. Bad idea.

A week later, I show up at Kanbayashi Onsen hot spring, weary from my overnight flight and long train journey to this remote part of Nagano. I am greeted with hot black bean tea and a friendly duty manager, and it all starts well. But then his expression changes to one of puzzlement.

"Where is your traveling companion?" he asks.

"It's just me," I reply.

"Oh."

It turns out I have paid about $323 for only a room in this hot-spring resort, based on two people sharing, even though there is only me. The price doesn't include any food, and it is too late to order any as the chef has already been informed of numbers. If you have ever been to a hot spring in Japan, you will know that one of the joys of the experience, once you have soaked your tired body, is to get dressed in a yukata *(cotton kimono) and tuck into a feast of carefully prepared local dishes. The food is half the point. No one books room-only at an* onsen.

"I'm so sorry. I could show you a nice rāmen place down the road," he offers, trying to help.

I am shattered. There is a foot of snow outside. And I am pretty sure that after a soak in a hot bath, I am not going to want to traipse down the road in the cold for a bowl of noodles, while everyone else enjoys a veritable feast in the hotel.

Of course, it is my fault. (Well, mine and Expedia's, for offering room-only places at an onsen.*) But knowing this doesn't help. The chatter begins in my head: Why couldn't you have just concentrated for five minutes and made the right booking in the first place? Why didn't you take the time to read the details? Typical. (Even though it's not actually typical at all. I'm usually pretty good at logistical stuff.) Sometimes the chaos just seems to take on a life of its own.*

But then my Japanese kicks in and I am full of apology. "Oh please don't worry, it's totally my fault. I should have paid better attention when

I made the booking. It's such a pity, as I was looking forward to delicious local Nagano food, but it's completely my fault for having messed up the arrangements. I am so sorry to cause you the embarrassment of this mix-up . . ."

There must be something about the tone of my voice when I speak Japanese, the extra-polite language it is only appropriate to use, and perhaps my body language, which mirrors that of the duty manager, gets him thinking. Perhaps it is the unexpectedly quiet response of the weary foreigner who just wants a hot bath and a tasty dinner, who is making no fuss and is, instead, apologizing profusely rather than being loud and brash, as visitors sometimes are, that makes him think twice.

"Please sit down and enjoy your tea and cake. I'll just pop into my office and see what I can do," he says, bowing and scuttling off.

He makes a phone call, and before I can finish the welcome snack, he is back with good news. He kneels beside me, apologizes again, and says that the chef will make a special exception as I have traveled so far, and I am welcome to have tonight's twelve-course meal on the house, if I would so care to partake of it. Would I ever! I am floored.

Humility and gentleness are met with humility and gentleness. No drama. No stress. Just kindness.

I thought about this as I tucked into my lotus root, shrimp, and green peas in miso in the hotel restaurant that evening. I mulled it over as I sent a silent prayer of gratitude for the chef who had so carefully prepared the deep-fried angelica spear with simmered burdock, earthy and woody with a spicy puff of smoke. While the Nagano beef and onions cooked over a candle in front of me, I considered why our natural response to a problem is so often to launch into a reaction of stress, anger, or blame. As I stirred in locally foraged mushrooms with my chopsticks, I thought about how those things rarely help to solve the problem.

And by the time the clam soup, local rice, and pickles arrived,

I had figured out three questions that can help us handle challenging situations in a calmer frame of mind. Next time you want to scream in a moment of conflict, take a deep breath, then ask yourself:

1. How do I really feel? What's the deeper feeling beneath the initial response of anger or frustration? Maybe it's actually about something else—loneliness, fear, guilt, or sadness, for example. This can help take the fire out of your initial response.

2. What's going on, and why is the person in front of me saying what they are saying? Listening carefully and trying to understand their point of view can help you understand, even if you don't agree. This can help you calm down and respond in a much more effective way.

3. What do I want to say and why do I feel I need to say it?

Is it because you want to find a way to find a resolution and move beyond the situation, or is it because your ego wants you to settle a score or win an argument? Focusing on a mutual resolution, instead of competition or manipulation, can allow you to deal with the situation more calmly and resolve it more quickly.

Try thinking about these questions the next time you feel anger rising, or you find yourself snapping at your children, your partner, or a colleague, and see if you can resolve things in a calmer way. Then notice how differently you feel when you have done that.

Try bringing your *wabi sabi* worldview to all of your relationships, and you'll soon notice how different they look with this perspective.

WABI SABI-INSPIRED WISDOM FOR NURTURING RELATIONSHIPS

- Wabi sabi *opens up a space for love.*
- *No one is perfect. Our connections deepen when we honor one another's imperfections.*
- *The four principles of the tea ceremony—harmony, respect, purity, and tranquility—can help us develop good relationships.*

TRY IT: CHANNELING THE SPIRIT OF THE TEA CEREMONY IN DAILY LIFE

Think of someone you are particularly close to—perhaps a spouse, a child, a parent, a friend, or a work colleague. Make a note of the ways in which you could apply the principles below in your day-to-day relationship with them. Your answers might be either emotional or practical suggestions.

❋ *Wa* (harmony)

- What could you do more of to encourage harmony?
- What could you do less of?
- What could you do differently?
- What could you try for the first time?
- What could you let go of, for the sake of harmony?
- What details of their life could you notice, and pay more attention to?
- What is that person's natural rhythm? How could you consider that more in your life together? (For example, timing of important conversations, giving them space after a long day, suggesting they sleep in after a hard week.)

- How could you help them consider *your* natural rhythm more in your life together?
- What could you share about yourself that would help them support you?

✳ *Kei* (respect)

- What do you respect about this person? How could you let them know about this?
- In what ways could you offer them kindness right now?
- In what ways could you show humility in your relationship with them?

✳ *Sei* (purity)

- When you look for the best in this person, what do you see?
- How could you let them know about this?
- Think back to the last time you had some kind of conflict with them. If you had approached it with a commitment to seeing the best in them, even in the middle of the conflict, what might have been different?
- List all the ways you care for this person. Find a lovely way to tell them.

✳ *Jaku* (tranquility)

- How could you nurture a sense of calm in your relationship?
- Are there particular times or scenarios where you tend to react in an emotionally charged way? How might you benefit from approaching a conflict situation with harmony, respect, purity, and tranquility? (It may not be easy, but it can make a huge difference.)
- How could you proactively build more space and peace into your time together?

人生行路

CHAPTER 7:
ENJOYING
THE CAREER
JOURNEY

can't imagine having a career conversation with a Japanese person in which the topic of *wabi sabi* comes up. The word "career" brings to mind striving, competition, pressure, a particular goal. *Wabi sabi* evokes pretty much the opposite of all those things. But having spent almost a decade helping people to shift to a career that lights them up or to find new ways to fall back in love with the one they already have, I can see that there is actually much we can learn by viewing our careers through the lens of *wabi sabi*.

That core teaching of *wabi sabi*—that everything is impermanent, imperfect, and incomplete—feels to me like a giant permission slip to explore and experiment within your career. Although we tend to think about a career as a linear thing, *wabi sabi* reminds us that life is cyclical and we can have more than one "career" in our lifetime. This chapter is all about how to enjoy the career *journey*, and that starts with understanding where you are right now, so you can choose how to move forward.

The virtuous cycle of perfect imperfection

The conflicting desires to fit in yet stand out, keep up and surge ahead, all in pursuit of an elusive perfection over there is a huge distraction from the life you already have over here.

In my work, I have come to realize just how influential the lure of perfection can be and not in a good way. It seeps into every area of people's lives, not least in their careers, crushing confidence and self-esteem and raising anxiety and stress levels. It also has a practical impact on how people allocate their precious resources—in particular, time and money.

The five main career scenarios that I come across in my work are:

1. "I love my job but find it too stressful. I'm not sure if I want a career change or a job change or just to find a better way of working."

2. "I hate my job, but I feel stuck (by a lack of self-confidence or ideas about what else I could do) or trapped (by circumstances, such as finances or commitments)."

3. "My job's okay and it pays the bills, but . . . [or "I am good at my job, but . . .] I dream of something else [very often something more creative], although the idea of actually doing it terrifies me."

4. "My main job recently has been parenting. I am planning to go back to work, but I need more flexibility in my working hours or arrangements, and I'm not sure my old job is even right for me anymore." Alternatively, "I am proud of the time I have spent raising my children, but I want something for myself now that they are older."

5. "I have been laid off and I cannot figure out whether it is a nightmare or a blessing in disguise."

In nearly all cases, what my clients think is the issue is rarely the actual issue. Lots of people cite money and time as their main challenges, but that is usually a matter of some smart prioritizing (and chapter 8 includes some tips to help you with that). It's also often the case that they are in the dark about just how many opportunities there are nowadays for flexible hours, telecommuting, or running our own businesses.

However, beneath all the resistance to change and the feelings of "stuckness," lies the real block: fear of not being good enough; fear of not knowing enough; fear of failure; fear of making a move without knowing how it will work out, fear of losing control (not that we are in control in the first place); fear of not being perfect. And although each person's situation is different, I have seen a pattern emerging—a vicious cycle of "failing at perfection," which looks something like this:

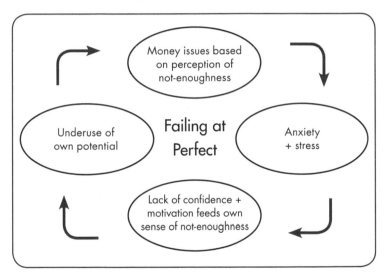

We can use all the *wabi sabi*–inspired wisdom and tools I have shared in this book to break this cycle, as we accept the idea of impermanence, imperfection, and incompleteness as the natural state of all things. But there is also a huge amount to be gained by simply relaxing, being gentler on ourselves, and making the choice to enjoy the journey.

Collectively, this can help us shift to a "perfectly imperfect" virtuous cycle like this:

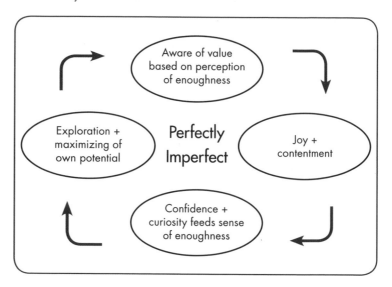

Use your *wabi sabi*–inspired tools

Whenever I am on a panel or run open forums for people in business, I am almost always asked a question related to competition, comparison, or enoughness. It's very hard to run a business with your eyes open and your ear to the ground and *not* find yourself comparing your "success" to the "success" of others.

This is also true in the world of salaried work. It's difficult to stay alert to what is going on in your workplace and your industry without running into situations that encourage comparison and competition. For as long as this helps you aspire to something you genuinely want, it can be helpful. But as soon as it detracts you from your own path, it can be damaging.

The thing to remember is this: someone else's success does not hinder your chances of achieving what you want. Their success may even open up new opportunities for you and others. They will walk their path; you are supposed to walk yours. You have everything you need to go wherever you want to go.

It's just as important to use your tools for nurturing relationships, reframing failure, and accepting your perfectly imperfect self at work as it is to use them in your life outside of work. If you show up with integrity and allow your inner beauty to shine, any workplace and any client will be lucky to have you. If they don't show you their appreciation, check in with your heart and see if it's time to move on.

The imperfect path your heart guides you along is the perfect path for you.

Look beneath the surface of your current career

Not long ago, I was in an external meeting where the icebreaker was: "If we take away your work, what else do we find?" One of the women there froze. You could see the dawning of a realization moving like a wave through her body. "Nothing. I am my work. And I didn't realize that until this moment. Oh wow, I wasn't expecting that. Something needs to change."

That woman is one of the most brilliant, inspiring, funny, and warm people I know. And yet she couldn't come up with anything to say about her life that wasn't connected with work. I happen to know that she has a half-finished manuscript tucked away in her desk, a deep love of travel, and a circle of lovely friends. But she had pushed all those things away in the pursuit of an elusive goal of career perfection, with the result that her work had moved in and swallowed up all the space. It had become all about what was on the surface—the achievements, the appraisals, the promotions, the salary and status, the mantle of busyness. She had, as do so many of us, forgotten that what lies beneath matters, too.

So let's take a moment to remind ourselves of those four emotional underlayers of Japanese beauty and see what happens if we layer them over our career paths:

Mono no aware
An awareness of the fleeting beauty of life.

1. What is good in your career right now?
2. Consider the life and career stage you are in and complete this sentence: "Now is the moment to . . ."
3. What do you need to do first in order to make the most of this moment?

Yūgen
The depth of the world as seen with our imagination. The beauty of mystery and of realizing we are a small part of something so much greater than ourselves.

1. How much are you trying to control the direction of your career path? What might happen if you let go a little and opened up to mystery?
2. What deeper purpose are you serving or could you serve with your career?
3. If you have untended dreams that have been shelved for too long, what kind of changes could you make to your working arrangements to give them some attention?

Wabi

The feeling generated by recognizing the beauty found in simplicity. The sense of quiet contentment found away from the trappings of a materialistic world.

1. How could you simplify your work life? How could you proactively reduce your workload and streamline communications to focus only on what really matters?
2. How could you minimize the drama, avoid the politics and gossip, and invite more calm into your working day?
3. If you are overworked due to your perfectionist tendencies, what space might open up for you if you trusted someone else with some of your work?
4. If you feel like you are just working to pay the bills, could you take a fresh look at your finances and figure out a way to live more simply, so the burden on your work is not so heavy?
5. Does your work come easily to you? In what ways are you using your natural talents? How could you do this more?

Sabi

A deep and tranquil beauty that emerges with the passage of time.

1. How has your career ripened over the years? What have you learned?
2. Are you trying to force your career too fast? What difference would it make if you relaxed into the rhythm of it, allowing the richness to build over time?
3. If you feel it's time for a change, what skills have you picked up that could serve you elsewhere? What have you learned

in the great school of life that could serve the next stage of
your career?

Just as these emotional elements of beauty are of great importance in Japanese aesthetics, they can be important guides on your
career path. They require pause, attention, tuning in, and being
open to wonder.

Life in contemporary Japan

For a period of more than two hundred years from the early
seventeenth century to the mid-nineteenth century, Japan was
virtually closed off from the world through a national isolationist
policy known as *sakoku*. This ended when Commodore Matthew
Perry and his famous "black ships" arrived in Tōkyō Bay from
America in 1853 and forced Japan to open to trade once again.
Within five years Japan had signed treaties with other countries
including the United Kingdom and Russia.

The influx of ideas and technology that followed had an
irreversible effect on the lifestyle of the Japanese. The country's
subsequent rise, post–World War II, from economic insignifi-
cance to world player, brought with it Westernization—Western
clothes, Western style, and, to some extent, Western thinking.
Since then, Japan has become a high-tech, high-earnings world.
The people have become affluent and a high standard of living
prevails. With this newfound wealth have come the rapid growth
of cities, a proliferation of skyscrapers, and the famous bullet train.

Even if you have never been to Japan, you probably have an
image of what working life looks like. Perhaps it involves suited
"salarymen" or the unfortunately named "OL" (office ladies),
packed into commuter trains by white-gloved station officials; or

exhausted workers nodding off on their journey home. Maybe the Japan in your mind's eye is the iconic image of pedestrians surging forward at Shibuya Crossing, under the glow of neon signs and giant screens—thousands of people with somewhere to be.

Tōkyō has an incredible energy, and millions of people *do* live this commuter life there, and in cities across Japan. I was one of them many moons ago, and there were aspects of it that I loved. But more than ever, as in so many places around the world, options are opening up for people who don't want to live and work in such a hurry anymore.

The slow revolution

Nestled deep in the mountains of Shimane Prefecture lies the charming town of Ōmori-chō. At its peak, a couple of centuries ago, the surrounding area of Iwami-Ginzan bustled with the energy of two hundred thousand people serving one of the world's largest silver mines. But when the mine closed in 1923, the town, like many former mining communities, slowly began to die. At one point, Ōmori-chō's population dwindled and might have disappeared completely had it not been for a huge local effort, including that of one pioneering couple, the Matsubas, who moved there in the early 1980s and helped breathe new life into the place. Now Iwami Ginzan is recognized as a beacon of sustainable development by UNESCO.[1]

Designer Tomi Matsuba and her husband, Daikichi, moved here nearly four decades ago with their young daughter. Ōmori-chō was Daikichi's hometown, and they thought the gentle pace of life would better suit their young family than Nagoya, where they lived. With few opportunities for work, Tomi began making patchworks from old fabrics, which her husband sold into retail stores. This was the humble beginning of a business that has gone on to become a leader in Japan's "slow clothing" scene,[2] with stores nationwide under the brand name Gungendō[3] (which takes its name from a Chinese word meaning "a place where everyone has their say"). Their company now employs around fifty local residents and many more in their stores nationwide.

Tomi told me:

> We do not see ourselves as a fashion brand. Increasing numbers of people share our values, and that is why they are drawn to our products. It is our mission to maintain the quality and heritage of all we offer, and to support people to live in a gentle and authentic way.

Besides using locally sourced natural materials and labor to produce their stylish clothing and housewares, Tomi and her husband have undertaken the renovation of several historic buildings, to preserve the history of the area. Overnight visitors are treated to some of Japan's finest traditional accommodation,[4] and a number of the buildings are used by the community for arts performances and exhibitions.

These days, if you take a stroll down Ōmori-chō's main street, you might see a group of young mothers chatting outside the bakery, a few people heading to work on their bicycles, or a couple of older friends on their way to pick mountain vegetables. You'll walk past rows of carefully maintained wooden houses and hear people calling gentle greetings to each other as they go about their day. This town is the embodiment of slow living, and there is a tangible sense of place and of pride in the community from those who call it home.

The life and career Tomi has built here has been a labor of love, and her work has evolved many times along the way. She is a pillar of the community, and can be proud of her role in bringing it back to life. There has been a particular influx of newcomers since the Great East Japan Earthquake in 2011, which prompted many people to reconsider the importance of material success and prioritize what really matters.

Not only are Tomi and her husband blazing a trail for sustainable business, they are also active as shining examples of how a career can be multifaceted and continually evolving. When they began, they had no idea where this adventure would take them. Now a grandmother, Tomi is still full of ideas and energy. Her life's work will never be done, and she is grateful for that.

Gungendō's mantra is "Life with roots." Tomi says, "Our ideal lifestyle is like that of a tree—putting down roots that spread through the land, standing firm and growing slowly. Enjoying our daily lives as we take root in the land, pursuing long-term goals, and having a positive influence on those around us."

Personally, I am particularly inspired by the fact that Tomi began Gungendō when she was forty-three, not much older than me as I write this. It's never too late to create something special. Tomi reminds us how a career can unfold to reveal a scattering of shining treasures, only evident when you surrender to the journey and follow your heart, adopting a career philosophy, not a single career goal.

Walk your own path

One of my favorite kanji in the Japanese language is the character 道, which means "path" or "road" when it is read as *michi*. But it is often used in combination with other characters to mean "the way," in which case it is read as *dō*. You may have heard of it: *Chadō* and *sadō* (different readings for 茶道) refer to "the way of tea," *bushidō* (武士道) is "the way of the warrior," and Japanese calligraphy is known as *shodō* (書道), "the way of writing." Among popular martial arts, we find *jūdō* (柔道), "the way of gentleness," and *karatedō* (空手道), often known outside Japan simply as karate, the "way of the empty hand."

In much the same way, our careers are paths. When we look back on the road we have walked thus far, we see that it is not just winding—it often goes back on itself; there are gentle curves and hairpin bends. Effort matters, and commitment is rewarded. The time it took to get to where we are is not the point. The time it will take us to get to where we will go next is not the point. In fact, the results themselves are not the point: the way you get to your results matters more than the results that you get.

Lessons from the dōjō

These days, you are more likely to find mixed-media artist Sara Kabariti in her painting studio than in the dōjō, but almost three decades on from her time spent training in martial arts in Japan, she says that the experience still informs her life on so many levels. "In a nutshell, I learned how to learn. I learned the importance of discipline, hard work, and persistence, but also approaching everything I do with great passion and joy. I spent many hundreds of hours practicing over and over, working on my form and strength."

NTC's Dictionary of Japan's Business Code Words, under the entry for *shūgyō* (修業, translated as "training for intuitive wisdom"), confirms this: "In the Japanese value system, the way things are done outweighs what is done. . . . The Japanese believe that the harder something is to learn and the more effort that is required to learn it, the more valuable the knowledge or the skill."[5]

In Japan, form is everything. This is true both in the handcrafting of items (which explains why artisans will take decades before they truly recognize their own skill) and in their attitude to life (which explains much of the formality and ritual in Japanese life). Potter Makiko Hastings described how she strives to improve the form of her craft without ever expecting to attain absolute perfection. She knows that imperfection is the true nature of things, so she works at edging closer to the best she can do and be, without a false expectation of where she will end up.

Excellence over perfection

When the notion of excellence is used as an aspirational motivator, it can be hugely valuable. This is in stark contrast to working toward an elusive goal of perfection with the expectation that we will "arrive," burning ourselves out as we relentlessly push on forward and ending up disappointed because the destination was never reachable in the first place. The difference in understanding is subtle, but the impact is immense.

This attention to form paid off for Sara Kabariti. Recalling the time she competed at the European *Jōdō* Championships,[6] she told me how the prospect of one particularly long *kata* (move) was making her really nervous. Her teacher came over and said, "Sara, after all your training, your body knows what to do, but your mind won't allow it to do it." At that moment, she understood and let go. She knew that we have to set intentions, show up to practice, do our best. And then trust. She and her partner went on to win the gold.

Sara says:

It's when we let go and trust that the magic really begins to happen. The Japanese are masters at finding the line of least resistance, even if it doesn't seem like the logical route. Martial arts teaches us to go with the flow of energy and motion, not against it. I also learned that the minute you think you either know it all or you think you cannot do it, you have lost it. I was shown early on to be open and fully in the present moment. Letting go is both a major life lesson and a daily practice. We can set intentions and show up for practice, but there comes a point where we have to trust and allow things to fall into place in good time. My mantra these days is "surrender."

Set your own pace

To make progress in the direction of your dreams, within the context of your perfectly imperfect life, you will need preparation, dedication, and trust in yourself and in the process. You have to let go of the need to have all the answers or a "perfect" picture of the future before playing your part in creating it. A *wabi sabi*–inspired worldview gives us permission to feel our way through life, paying less attention to what we think others think (or what we think we should do based on what others think) and more attention to what really matters to us. Keep asking questions and keep moving, sometimes slowly, sometimes quickly, depending on the ebb and flow of life.

In reading *Nihonjin no kokoro, tsutaemasu*, a short book about the world of tea by former *iemoto* (head) of the Urasenke school of tea, Sen Genshitsu, I came across the word *johakyū* (序破急). This refers to three different speeds of action—slow, a little faster, and fast.[7] Sen Genshitsu explained how there is a tempo to the tea ceremony and practitioners must vary the speed as required. He went on to say how they must vary their effort level, too—sometimes being gentle, sometimes adding a little strength, sometimes really going for it. As he concluded, this can also be great advice for life.

I have talked a fair bit about slowing down to allow yourself to notice more, sense more, see more, and experience more. This comes from a starting point of rushing, which seems to be the default pace for so many of us these days. But slowing down doesn't mean calling time on a desire to do meaningful work in the world or having ambition or getting involved in exciting things. Slowing down is important as a counterpoint to running fast, and sometimes it's good to vary the pace.

And just as Sen Genshitsu said, varying our effort levels is vital for our well-being, too. We cannot give any project, meeting, opportunity, or conversation our full attention when we are trying to juggle many things at once. We have to prioritize well, get organized, and focus on one thing at a time.

We have to put our effort where it is going to have the greatest impact, and take us in a direction we actually want to travel in. And for every time we give something our everything, we have to put other things to one side. After a major effort, we have to build in recovery time and give ourselves permission to take it easy for a while. Using these three gears of speed and three gears of effort can make all the difference to whether or not we enjoy our career journeys and stay well along the way.

Being open to change

The world of work is changing at the fastest pace since the Industrial Revolution. Many traditional job roles are disappearing and new opportunities are opening up. None of us can know what a career will look like fifty years from now. We can try to hold on to how things are or we can embrace the evolution, making the most of it to carve out a career that supports the kind of life we want to live.

This statement has never been truer, when rapidly evolving technology has given many of us the option to work from anywhere, to any rhythm we choose. More than ever, we have to recognize that even if we don't change, the working world will. The impact on our careers will be determined by whether we embrace that or try to hold on to the status quo, even as the status quo is shifting.

Our skill sets are not usually industry specific and can serve us in many ways. When we relax into the knowledge that our careers are dynamic, not static, we open ourselves up to unknown possibilities. Recognizing and planning for the impermanence of the jobs we once thought were secure makes us better prepared if changes are imposed upon us, and reminds us that if we are having a hard time, we don't have to do it forever. Would we even want to? We are likely to want very different things at twenty, forty, sixty, and eighty years of age.

There is no single perfect career path. There is only the one that we are constructing as we go.

All of this goes against everything many of us have been taught about how to be successful—that we should follow one path and stick to it, that money and status are the goal, that if you don't reach some particular image of perfection you have failed. Having spent most of the past decade helping people shift between careers, start their own businesses, or reprioritize to do more of what they love, I know that attitudes are slowly shifting, but we have a long way to go. On the whole, from what I have seen in my work, we still care far too much about what other people might think and don't pay enough attention to what makes sense for us.

We increasingly need to be able to see, read, empathize, question, adapt, and course-adjust to accommodate this transitioning world of work. Experts tell us that some of us, and likely many of our children, will live to one hundred and beyond.[8] What difference would it make if you knew that this was going to be true for you?

Questions for looking at the long view

- What difference would it make if you knew you would be likely to be working well into your seventies or even your eighties?
- Do you want to be doing what you are doing now until then, presuming that kind of work still exists?
- If not, what kind of work might suit you later in life?
- What difference would it make if you knew that your current career would have its moment and then fade, to make way for another?
- Would you have a different approach to your current role?
- What skills or training might you explore?
- Would you give your creative ideas or side business more attention?
- What else would you nurture?

Now, ask yourself those questions again, but this time instead of looking for the logical answers, tell me this: What does your heart say?

Remember, your heart's response to beauty is the essence of *wabi sabi*. So what kind of beauty could you create with your career?

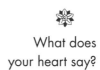

What does your heart say?

Ask the kind of questions that prompt inspired answers

When we ask children "What do you want to be when you grow up?" we are usually trying to sow the seeds of dreams. But then we sometimes respond in a way that crushes those dreams and can cause long-term damage. "An artist? Oh no, dear, you don't want to be an artist. You can't make money doing that." Or children end up attaching their dreams to a specific job they think will make us proud, in many cases the same job they see us doing. It's what they know, or what they think we'd like them to do, or what we keep telling them we think they *should* do.

But then what if they don't make it into that profession? Or if they do make it and don't like it, but don't want to leave because they feel like they'd be letting us down? Or if they get caught up in a cycle of hustling and jostling for position, status, clients, salary, and recognition and, before they know it, they are in midlife, burned out and wondering what happened to the past twenty years? I'm pretty sure none of us wants that for our children or, indeed, for ourselves.

All of these are examples of things I have seen happen time and again to real people in my community. People come to us for support in discovering how to do what they love because they can no longer stand to do what they are doing, but don't know how to change or figure out what else they could do. The good news is they have no idea just how vast the possibilities are.

A recent international report on the future of work, based on surveys of more than ten thousand people across Asia, the UK, and the United States stated: "We are living through a fundamental transformation in the way we work. Automation and 'thinking machines' are replacing human tasks and jobs, and changing the skills that organisations are looking for in their people."[9]

As part of the same report, Blair Sheppard, global leader of strategy and leadership development at PwC said: "So what should we tell our children? That to stay ahead, you need to focus on your ability to continually adapt, engage with others in that process, and most importantly retain your core sense of identity and values."[10]

Questions we can ask to invite a different kind of career journey

- What inspires you?
- What matters to you?
- What would you like to create?
- What would you like to change?
- What would you like to experience?
- How could you help people?
- What kind of place would you like to work in?
- What kind of people would you like to work with?
- How would you like to spend your days?
- How do you want to feel about your work?
- What assumptions are you making about your opportunities that may not be true?

It bears repeating: there is no single way to live your life; there is no single career path; there is no perfect way to build your career. There is only evolving it, and it's up to you if you choose to do that in a way that brings you delight.

The waking dream

There's something about Japan that has always made me feel that anything is possible. Even back when I couldn't read any signs, hardly knew anyone, and could barely hold a conversation, I always felt something in the air that gave me an extra boost . . . of what, I'm not quite sure. But that "something" made me open and curious, and led me to all sorts of experiences I could never have imagined, from life-altering encounters with random strangers to hosting my own TV show. In some ways, it felt like a waking dream. Even now, when I return, it often still does.

I want to gift you some of that, wrapped up like a treasure in a *furoshiki* cloth,[11] to offer you inspiration and nourishment on your career path. Every time your dreams seem to be disappearing to the periphery of your life, untie the *furoshiki* and inhale a little of the magic. Take a moment to bring your dream into your field of vision, then bring yourself back to the present and feel your way to the next step on your path. Ask yourself what is the one thing you could do right now, to take you closer to that dream? What does your heart say?

We cannot know the timeline. We cannot predict the path. But we can be intentional in our steps and pause once in a while to experience the beauty all around.

> 日々是好日 (*nichinichi kore kōnichi*)
> Every day is a good day.
>
> —*Zen proverb*[12]

WABI SABI–INSPIRED WISDOM
FOR ENJOYING THE CAREER JOURNEY

- *There is no one perfect career path.*
- *Your path may contain several different careers, each supporting your priorities, as you move through the cycle of your life.*
- *The way you get to your results matters more than the results that you get.*

TRY IT: EXPLORE YOUR PATH

First, in a notebook, answer these questions:

❋ What jobs or roles have you had, either paid or unpaid, that taught you something? (Make a list.) What did each teach you?

❋ What have you studied at any level that you found interesting? This can be anything where you have spent time to learn about something in depth, formally or informally.

❋ What other major experiences have you had?

❋ What particular moments of fleeting beauty stand out in your memory?

Next, on a double page, draw a horizontal timeline, with vertical lines to mark each decade (or every five years if you are under thirty). Looking at your answers to the above questions, map out the most important experiences so far in your life. Mark any points when you had an "aha" moment.

Now draw lines between the things that are connected in some way. What had to happen for something else to happen? What themes can you see?

Now, with all the information in front of you, answer these questions:

❋ What have been the most important career decisions affecting your happiness along the way?

❋ What or who are you particularly grateful for on your career path to date?

❋ What do you need right now?

❋ What is one thing you could do to step into the next phase of your career with intention and trust, whether that is deepening what you do or moving in a new direction?

今を生きる

CHAPTER 8:
CHERISHING THE
MOMENTS

N ight has fallen, and I am running a little late. Clutching a bottle of wine I can't really afford, I stare wide-eyed at the shrine gate ahead of me. I am actually here. Pinching myself, I pass through the gate and turn left to the rambling, old house, known by the shrine name Tenmangū. The low hum of excited chatter floats through the air, mingling with the gentle croaking of a hundred frogs. I think about the gathered guests and almost turn to leave. At nineteen, I am intimidated by the prospect of a room full of Japan scholars, linguists, art dealers, and other people with far more knowledge on just about everything than me. And I don't know a soul.

But then I remember what brought me here. How Lost Japan, a wonderful book written by the owner of this house, encouraged me through my high school exams, promising mystery and adventure, if only I could get into college. How every time I struggled to write another essay, I picked up the book, read a couple of pages, and was inspired to do one more hour.

On arrival in Kyōto, I sent a note to thank the author, Alex Kerr, longtime Japan resident and now one of the country's most famous cultural observers. To my surprise, I received a letter back from his assistant, inviting me to this party at his home, one of the enchanting places I read about in Lost Japan.

The house and the company do not disappoint. I spend most of the evening observing fascinating conversations about East Asian history, politics, antiques, and all sorts of other things I feel unqualified to talk about. But just being here, in this centuries-old house, in among it all, is *enough. At one point we are invited into the old* doma, *or kitchen area, now used as a writing studio. Somehow everything in this space, open to the rafters, seems magnified. A giant sheet of mulberry paper has been spread out on the long table and, huge brush in hand, Alex Kerr is doing some of the most beautiful calligraphy I have ever seen.*

Time slows. Voices soften. People seem to be frozen in position, smiles on their faces, candlelight throwing shadows across the room. I think, This moment is special. Tuck it inside your pocket of treasures for safekeeping.

A couple of decades on, many details of that day are blurry, but that moment, which I chose to keep as a precious treasure, remains as clear as if it were yesterday.

The real kind of perfect

I'll let you in on a secret. "Perfect" is actually one my favorite words. I use it all the time, but only ever in the context of moments. I believe that is the only occasion perfection is real. The tiniest slice of time can hover, shimmering, in momentary stillness. And then it is gone. A perfect moment in an imperfect world.

That moment in Alex Kerr's studio at Tenmangū was perfect. The moment I sat in my hospital bed looking out over the sea, holding my precious newborn baby to my chest as the sun rose, knowing that this second child would be my last, was perfect. The moment this morning, when I exchanged an unspoken word with a sparrow looking in on me at my writing desk, was perfect.

In a world constantly in flux, moments like this can feel as if time itself is winking at us. For an instant we find ourselves completely immersed in the experience, not bothered about the past or future while simultaneously being aware that the moment itself will not last. In literature this is sometimes called "a haiku moment," a description that captures the poetic beauty of beholding such a delicious sliver of experience.

These kinds of treasures are to be found in the smallest details of daily life, if we can slow down, be present, and pay attention long enough to notice. In that single heartbeat before the bird flew away, *wabi sabi* was present, as I experienced a natural beauty even more exquisite for its imminent vanishing.

The call of beauty

Wabi sabi is a gentle gauge of exquisite moments.

One lady in her seventies told me, "I feel *wabi sabi* when I'm in a space alone but can sense the lingering comforting presence of people who were there until a moment ago."

It is the anticipation of a loved one's return, just before the airport's arrivals doors open. A campfire story sent into the smoky air. The memory of a kiss, while you are still kissing.

When we look back on our lives, these are the kinds of moments that we remember. When we rush too fast, eyes locked somewhere on the future, or staring at our smartphones, or distracted by someone else's path, we miss the opportunity to stop and collect our own moments of beauty and to sense *wabi sabi*.

We know how delightful life can be when we are present to it and yet we still spend our days rushing, distracted, stressed out, boxed in, on track for a life that doesn't quite feel like ours. When we truly open our eyes and hearts, beauty calls to us, through the chaos and the noise. It shows us a fleeting glimpse of the version of our lives where our soul is singing because we harnessed our talents, gave attention to our ideas, nurtured our love, and really showed up for life.

Sometimes we feel this but turn away from it because it doesn't look how we expected it to look. It's not the shiny, polished life we have been taught to desire: the perfect house, job, car, partner, family, or whatever. But when we are present and really listen for the call of beauty, we discover the life that was meant for us. Our perfectly imperfect life.

Beauty calls quietly. We have to be perceptive to its signal and then play our part. The creative urge, the pull to a rural life, the yearning for friendships that go deeper—whatever it is that is calling you to a particular kind of beauty, heed that call, for it is the beauty of life itself.

Live long, live well

According to UNDP, Japan has the highest life expectancy of any country in the world,[1] with 67,824 centenarians alive in 2017.[2] Within Japan, the rural village of Matsukawa in Nagano has the highest life expectancy of anywhere.[3]

When this was announced by the Ministry of Health, Labour and Welfare, the mayor of Matsukawa, Akito Hirabayashi, said in an interview:

> I was bowled over to hear this news. It's not that we have done anything special to achieve this. We are blessed with a beautiful natural environment, many people work daily in the fields and we eat food that we have grown ourselves. There is also a strong sense of community, and I am sure all these things have contributed.[4]

A friend of mine who visited Matsukawa to cover this for TV said, "I saw many local people out walking, exercising together in parks, and swimming. They also have a lot of cooking lessons, and there was a general sense of positivity in the town." The local government investigated further and found three main reasons for the high life expectancy: a high standard of public health, a high level of health awareness and participation in health-building activities, and a meaningful life with high motivation for work and participation in social activities.[5]

It's not just about living long. It's also about living well. And *wabi sabi* is a barometer of well-being.

Ayumi Nagata, a young shop assistant, told me:

> When we are so busy that we no longer sense *wabi sabi*, we know that we have gone offtrack. It's a reminder to slow down, breathe, and take time to find beauty. When we can't sense *wabi sabi*, we are distracted, or under pressure, or we aren't taking care of ourselves.

When we look back on our lives, what do we want to remember? How do we want to feel? What do we want to have contributed? What will have made our life meaningful? How many moments of beauty do we want to have experienced along the way?

And let's not forget that there is beauty in every emotion. The more we allow ourselves to feel, the closer we get to that ravishing sense of aliveness and awe, even in the midst of challenging experiences.

Remember, one of the most fundamental teachings of *wabi sabi* is that we are impermanent, just like everyone we love and everything in the world around us. We will not live forever. We may not even live a long time. Life is precious and fleeting. It's up to us to make the most of it at each stage, starting where we are right now.

Lessons from an elder

I love talking to older people, hearing stories about the past and getting their perspective on today's world. It was, therefore, a real pleasure to spend an afternoon with Mineyo Kanie, the ninety-four-year-old daughter of the late Gin-*san*, at her home in Nagoya. Gin-*san* and her twin sister, Kin-*san*, were known for being the world's oldest identical twins, living to 108 and 107 respectively. Full of fun and vitality, they were frequently featured on television and became national celebrities in Japan. I wanted to know what Kanie-*san* had learned from her mother and aunt about living a good long life. I was also interested to hear the perspective of someone who, statistically, is very likely to live to a ripe old age herself.

Kneeling on a flat cushion in her tatami-matted lounge, Kanie-san exudes a gentle calm. You get the sense that she has seen it all. When she was born, in this very house, there was nothing but rice fields as far as the eye could see. Now it is a residential neighborhood in the bustling city of Nagoya.

Over green tea and blueberry pastries, we chat about parenting and politics, society and friendship. We laugh a lot. Her cheeky giggle is infectious. At one point, Kanie-san looks wistfully off into the distance and says, "You know, getting old is fine, but it's sad when hardly any of your friends are left."

We are meeting just before the annual Hina-Matsuri *Girls' Day celebration, when people traditionally display a set of ornamental dolls dressed as the emperor and empress, attendants, and musicians in the traditional dress of the Heian period (794–1185). The display in Kanie-san's living room instead features two dolls dressed as Kin-san and Gin-san, whose names meant "gold" and "silver" respectively, a gift from a fan many years ago. Occasions like this mark the passage of time, in a similar way to the seasons. It's a reminder to gather with loved ones and to celebrate life.*

Besides honoring tradition, Kanie-san also puts much store by simple daily rituals and having a routine to keep her active. She makes her own meals from scratch, always from natural ingredients, often using food she has grown herself. Full of energy, Kanie-san regularly cycles a short way to pay her respects at her family's grave, and tends her garden daily. On a practical note, she uses small plates for her meals and stops eating before she feels full. In Japan they call this hara hachi bu *(腹八分), putting your chopsticks down when your stomach is 80 percent full.*

Kanie-san *tells me, "We don't need much to live a good life. When you are grateful for what you do have, and share it with those you love, whatever else you need comes." Her deep appreciation of the gifts of a simple life is* wabi sabi *personified. She goes on: "Don't waste energy worrying about what you don't have. That is the route to misery. Instead, pay attention to the good already present in your life, and do your best at whatever you are doing. There is joy in the satisfaction of that."*

"Stay cheerful. Don't worry so much about things that don't really matter."

Perhaps Kanie-san's most important advice is this:

Pondering your own longevity

In chapter 7, we considered the potential effect on your career of living to one hundred, but what about if you actually have a much shorter life than you expected? Let's take a second look at different scenarios:

- What difference would it make to your current work, long-term finances, and priorities if you knew you were going to live for ten more years? For only one more year?
- What might your end-of-life self think about how you are living right now?

- What advice might your end-of-life self give to your current self?

Imagining different possibilities for the one thing we cannot know—how long we will live—can be an enlightening tool for discovering what really matters to us and reprioritizing accordingly. It can help us to reconsider what is truly urgent in our lives, and reveal how many of the things we thought were urgent really are not. It can inspire us to make the most of now and step away from the daily hustle to breathe deeply and soak it all up.

Lessons from the airport

I am at the airport, waiting for a flight to Tōkyō, holding a jar of expensive face cream in each hand. I'm trying to decide between the two because if I buy one, I'll get something else for free. And then I realize: It's happening. I have caught myself in the act of being dazzled by the shiny thing and lured by the promise of softer skin and fewer wrinkles, while I'm waiting for a flight to Japan to research the concept of beauty in imperfection. As the irony dawns, I laugh out loud, put the containers back on the shelf, and save myself fifty dollars.

My willingness to spend money on "antiaging" cream is an indication of my resistance to the natural aging process of my own body. And I am not alone. The antiaging beauty industry has global sales of close to \$300 billion a year.[6] That is one hundred times the global spending on tackling and treating malaria.[7]

We are so obsessed with trying to hang on to our youth that we have forgotten to look for our own *sabi* beauty.

The beauty of aging

It is a chilly December morning and I rise early to have breakfast with my old friend Duncan Flett, who has lived in Kyōto for almost twenty years. Duncan is a hugely knowledgeable tour guide who has his finger on the pulse of the old city. He has recommended we meet at the pop-up Kishin Kitchen, which unbeknownst to us, will soon be given the honor of "The Best Breakfast in Japan."[8] The name "Kishin," written 喜心, means "joyful heart," and you can tell that every part of our breakfast has been prepared by chefs who truly love their work. During the meal, ably hosted by the talented young Toshinao Iwaki, we are served rice three times. The first helping, carefully placed in a handcrafted ceramic bowl, is offered just after it has finished cooking and is shiny, steaming, and sticky. Not long after, once it has been allowed to rest a little, we are offered another serving. And then, toward the end of our breakfast, our bowls are refilled with the okoge—the "honorable burnt bits" from around the edges of the pan.

The rice is delicious at every stage of cooking. There are highlights each time—the freshness of the first helping, the familiarity of the second, and the texture of the third. My favorite is actually the okoge, *the final stage of the rice, but the chef can only get to the* okoge *by taking the rice through the earlier stages of cooking first. It gets better with time.*

We have a tendency to look at the aging process as something to be avoided, feared even. But everything about *wabi sabi* tells us that it is to be embraced—that we bloom and ripen with time; that our character develops and our wisdom deepens as we age; that we have more to offer the world with every experience we go through.

If you think about who you truly admire, it's likely that you will include someone older than you in your list. And yet we find it hard to see the value of aging in ourselves. We spend valuable time and money trying to cling to our youth on the surface while ignoring the beauty and wisdom of age underneath.

Reverend Takafumi Kawakami, deputy head priest of the Shunkō-in Temple in Kyōto, told me:

Wabi sabi reminds us to embrace each life stage, so we can age with grace.

If you look at the *wabi sabi* concept, you see an aging process. This is connected to the Buddhist concept of *mujō*, impermanence. I was recently on a panel of global-health experts where everyone was discussing how to keep ourselves younger for longer, as if we have forgotten that aging is part of the natural cycle of life. We fear getting older. We fear dying. We want to hold on to our youth and our own existence for as long as possible. But *wabi sabi* teaches us to enjoy the aging process and to relax into it as the most natural of things. It's okay to get old. We are supposed to get old. It's okay to know we are not going to be here forever because that helps us treasure the time we do have, and find virtue or meaning in our lives.

Wabi sabi encourages us to choose the path of serenity and contentment by accepting where we are in the natural cycle of our life. Using the tools I have shared in this book, we can turn away from stress and drama and release the aggressive energy of the hustle to make way for the nourishing energy of the flow.

Transitioning between life stages can be difficult, especially if we don't acknowledge or accept what is happening to our bodies, minds, and emotions. It is often in our times of major transition that things feel harder, more confusing, scary even, but also, it is in those times that we can see tremendous growth and flourishing. Sometimes we wait until something major happens to kick us from one life stage to another, but we don't have to.

If we are open to the transition, instead of holding on too tight to what has been, we can experience great insights and flow into the next stage, whether or not we feel ready. In this way, *wabi sabi* can remind us to live mindfully, taking each stage as it comes, growing into our wisdom, and taking care of ourselves along the way.

The Japanese use the word *fushime* (節目), which means "the node on a bamboo shoot," to acknowledge that we grow in stages and to describe important moments of transition in our lives. These times of transition are often celebrated with ceremonies and words of thanks to the people who have supported a person through that particular life stage. I think it is a lovely way to recognize that simply making the transition from one life stage to another is something worth celebrating together.

When we opt to live at a pace that suits us, doing the best we can and accepting that is all we need to do, everything feels different. Each stage of life is a time for growth. We are always learning and changing, whether we actively participate in that or not. At any time, whether things are flowing or tough, we can ask ourselves questions such as:

- What can I learn here?
- How am I growing right now?
- What change can I see or feel, inside or out?
- What do I need to let go of to move into my next life stage?
- How can I better take care of myself right now?

This brings our attention back into the experience of our lives as they are happening, and helps us to ease ourselves into the next stage. And when we fully embrace life, at whatever age, that's when our inner beauty shines through.

Finding joy in small things

Without exception, all the older people I spoke to in researching this book talked about the importance of finding beauty in everyday life. We can do this simply by slowing down and looking for things to appreciate: watering flowers, baking cakes, watching the sunset, counting the stars, reading a poem, taking a walk, making something. Even chores can be a meditation if we choose to make them so.

We can create rituals to bring us into the present. Before I sit down to write, I boil the water for tea and ponder the *Hamlet* quote on my favorite mug: "To thine own self be true." This is my writing ritual. It reminds me that I am investing time in something that I care about. And it makes the tea taste better.

We can also be open to the unexpected. My memories of travels in Japan are punctuated with the kindness of strangers: the day I went cycling through the fields of Okayama and an old woman stopped me to offer a freshly harvested watermelon, so big it would only just fit in my basket; the government official who arranged my forest-bathing session and gave up his Saturday morning to chauffeur me to the woods; the countless times I have been lost and people have accompanied me all the way to

 my destination. Each of these has brought joy, and I have tried every time to pay it forward, **Small moments** which brings another kind of joy, when you **matter.** can help someone else.

Perfectly imperfect planning

Accepting that everything is imperfect, impermanent, and incomplete is not an excuse to throw caution to the wind and avoid any kind of planning. For me, the opposite is true. Smart scheduling can help us prioritize what really matters, make more space in our lives for experiencing beauty, and ensure we are making the most of our lives.

HOW TO PLAN FOR MORE PERFECT MOMENTS

A well-lived life is a constant dance between dreaming and doing. The important thing here is not to obsess about perfect planning. You cannot know what is around the corner, so overplanning can lead to unnecessary stress when things change. It's about making a few key decisions so you don't lose your days to the whims of others.

Part A: the brain dump

You will need: sticky notes, several large sheets of paper, and a pen.

1. Gather every single notebook/diary/list/note/reminder that is currently active as a way of reminding you to do things.

2. On several large sheets of paper, write a heading for each of the key areas of your life: Family, Work, Hobbies, Health, Friends, Finances, Home, etc.

3. Go through each of your to-do lists/reminders/diary/ notebooks in turn and write one item you need "to do" on one sticky note, then stick it under the most relevant area. Repeat this for every single item on every single one of your to-do lists/reminders, writing down any and every task that requires time and attention from you. This may take a while.

4. When you've finished, make some notes about which areas of your life have the most to-do items. What does that tell you? Are there any surprises?

Part B: the possibilities

Now imagine your life five years from now, at a point where you feel contented and inspired. (We cannot know the timeline of any of our dreams, but this exercise can help make important decisions to take you in their direction.) Make notes using the following prompts:

- How old are you?

- Where are you living?

- What are you doing?

- What do you look forward to each day?

- When things are going really well, how do you feel?

- What are you grateful for?

Part C: the shift

In order to make that dream a possibility, change is inevitable. Use the questions below to help you identify what kind of changes might be involved:

- What needs to be different by this time next year in order for that dream to be even a remote possibility several years from now?

- How would you like to describe yourself a year from now?

- How would you like to describe your home a year from now?

- How would you like to describe your work life a year from now?

- How would you like to describe your finances a year from now?

- What would you like to have created a year from now?

Part D: the prioritizing

In my experience, the single-most important shift you can make to soulfully simplify your schedule is to think in terms of projects, not tasks. A project is something that has a defined beginning and end. An example might be "Career Change Project," "Write My Book Project," or "Wedding Project." It is a way of focusing your attention on something that really matters to you. Choose a maximum of five projects that you want to bring to life in the next twelve months. You don't have to start them all at the same time, and they can be spread over the twelve months.

Part E: the realignment

Now get five fresh pieces of paper and write each of your projects as the heading this time. Go back to your sticky notes and reallocate them onto your project sheets. You may be shocked at how many sticky notes you have left unassigned, showing just how committed you are to things that have nothing to do with the life you want to be living.

Part F: a new way of planning

Make a plan to finish, delegate, or forget about any of the to-do items that do not fit with your principal projects. For ongoing household chores and other such responsibilities, it can help to bundle them and then go through them all at once.

For example, in my house we deal with all our household finances twice a month.

Then revise your weekly schedule to ensure that you are spending a significant amount of your time working on the projects that really matter to you. Instead of trying to squeeze your dreams in around the edges, diarize your projects first, then plan everything else around them.[9]

Soulful simplicity in your finances

Every time we worry about money, expend energy feeling resentful about something we cannot afford, or regret something we bought that we didn't really need, we pull ourselves away from the here and now. Being anxious or distracted hampers our ability to feel *wabi sabi* and experience beauty. It may seem an unlikely connection, but some degree of financial planning and money management can make a huge difference to how present we can be in our lives, and consequently how we make the most of them.

My first year in Japan was spent living with a homestay family. My homestay mother—*Okāsan*, as I called her—taught me everything about managing household finances. She had a part-time job comparing prices for supermarkets, before the days of price-comparison technology and online grocery shopping. She carried this savvy into her own household management and had immaculate *kakeibo* (journals for household accounts), filled with columns of numbers. She was aware of every yen that came in and out of her house. In Japan, *kakeibo* have been popular for almost a century. These days, the top *kakeibo* app, Zaim, invented by a woman named Takako Kansai on her commute to work, has more than seven million users.

I would often find *Okāsan* at the kitchen table, feeding *chikuwa* (processed fish sticks) to the dog with one hand and flipping through the newspaper with the other, searching for money-off coupons. She never did more than a basket of shopping at a time, always waiting until the end of the day to get the bargains.

At the time, as a student on the other side of the world from home, I was living on a very tight budget. My room and board were covered, but the rest was up to me. At the beginning of each month, I would buy a batch of bus tickets for the rainy days when I couldn't cycle to school, put a little aside for my exploration fund, and then go to the bank for a pile of ¥100 coins. I would stack these up in piles of four and tape them together, one pile for each lunchtime. A coffee in a local *kissaten* (coffee shop) would set you back around ¥250, so ¥400 was not much of a budget for lunch. It would stretch to a bowl of rice and some soup, or a bag of raisin buns from the shop across from our classroom. Sometimes I'd sacrifice my lunch for a new pen or some cute stickers, Japanese stationery being a guilty pleasure of mine that remains to this day.

What I learned from my Japanese *Okāsan* was the importance of clarity, priority, and practice around finances. Keeping a *kakeibo* of my income and expenditure helped me understand what I had access to. I also kept notes of my savings, so I always knew where I was. I prioritized what mattered to me (getting to school, having adventures, and lunch/stationery, mostly in that order). And then I made it a habit, checking in weekly. These are habits I have carried with me ever since, and I still keep my own version of a *kakeibo* to this day.

Mindful spending.
Mindful saving.
Mindful living.

DECLUTTERING FINANCES

To declutter your finances in a soulfully simple way, ask yourself these questions:*

Clarity

- What exactly is coming in?

- What exactly is going out? Where is it going?

- What are your net assets? (In the broadest terms, this is the salable value of everything significant you own, including savings and investments, minus everything you owe.) If you are in a long-term relationship, what is your shared position?

- Are there any places you have been spending money based on a vision of an elusive "perfect life," which you no longer feel the need to chase?

- How do you feel about what you have discovered?

Whatever you discover, remember, you are where you are. Use your self-acceptance tools from chapter 4 (see page 104) to respond to any feelings of regret or anxiety that arise based on how you have been spending money. What matters is what you do next.

---

* These questions are intended to give you a fresh perspective on your finances. Please seek the support of a professional debt counselor or financial adviser if necessary.

Priority

- What do you really value?

- What are you actively prioritizing in the way you are using your money? Does this fit with what you value? If not, what do you need to change?

- Where are you spending money on things you don't really care about? What's stopping you from cutting out this expenditure altogether?

- How could you better use your money as a tool to invest in your current and future well-being and happiness?

Practice

- What do you need to change to make this happen?

- How can you make this part of your daily, weekly, or monthly routine so that mindful spending and saving become a habit?

When you have true clarity around your financial situation, and make financial decisions and plans based on what really matters to you and your family, you can reduce or remove three major sources of stress:

- Future regret about things you buy but don't need
- Future resentment about things you can't afford *because* of the things you bought that you don't need
- Worry about how you will afford to support yourself and your family in the future

This makes room for you to carve out your own perfectly imperfect life and frees you up to look for happiness right where you are.

WABI SABI–INSPIRED WISDOM
FOR CHERISHING THE MOMENTS

- *Embracing each life stage allows you to age with grace.*
- *You will not be here forever. Neither will your loved ones. Make the most of one another and of each day.*
- *The only true perfection is found in fleeting moments of beauty. Cherish each one.*

TRY IT: NOTICING ALL THE THINGS

A millennium ago, in her famous publication, *The Pillow Book*, Japanese poetess Sei Shōnagon wrote many artful lists of "Things That . . ." (for example, "Things That Do Not Linger") as a way of noticing the world around her and cherishing precious moments. Inspired by this, make your own lists or poems, using the following prompts or making up your own:

❀   Things I Only Notice When I Close My Eyes

❀   Things I Want to Keep in My Pocket of Treasures

❀   Things That Make My Heart Expand

結びに

AFTERWORD: TYING IT ALL TOGETHER

t's early March now, and I am sitting outside a café on the Philosopher's Path in Kyōto. I have a hot coffee in one hand and a blanket tucked around my knees. Somewhere, a wind chime is tinkling, and the few remaining green leaves are shivering on the branches of trees alongside the waterway. A few weeks from now the cherry blossom will burst forth and this path will be full of tourists. But for now I have it to myself.

I am reflecting on the conversation I had a moment ago with Hiraiwa-san, a young woman who works in the elegant Ginishō homewares shop just along the way, owned by KisoArtech, an innovative architecture company from Nagano. I asked her why she thought customers might sense an air of *wabi sabi* in her shop, where the walls are mottled, the small-batch items are all honed by hand from local wood, and the colors are sublimely dark and thoughtful. Her answer had nothing to do with any of those things.

She said, "I think it's because we are in a place where we experience the changing seasons intimately, and there is a blurred boundary between inside and out, with the shop set just on the edge of the waterway. It feels like we are part of nature here."

I have probably been to this part of Kyōto more than fifty times, first as a teenager, for weekly ikebana lessons at Mrs. Tanaka's house nearby and, more recently, seeking out fireflies on summer evening cycles with Mr. K. Once, as a penniless student, I took a lonely winter walk trying to figure out how to stretch my meager budget for the rest of the month. Another time there was tea and cake in the autumn. And now *here I am again, at the turn of the season, reflecting on how far we have traveled and all that we have learned in our search for the truth about* wabi sabi.

What started out as an exploration into beauty became so much more than that. It became a whole new way of experiencing the world, not with the logical mind but with the feeling heart, and with all our senses. *Wabi sabi* has shown us how fleeting moments of exquisite, evanescent beauty can remind us of the preciousness of life itself.

> *A small bowl sitting in one's hand*
> *Contains the whole of the universe.*[1]
>
> —RAKU KICHIZAEMON XV,
> FIFTEENTH-GENERATION JAPANESE POTTER

For me, the greatest teaching of *wabi sabi* has been the shift in perspective. Looking at the world through the lens of *wabi sabi* has transformed it into a more beautiful, gentle, and forgiving place, full of possibility and delight.

Early on in this book I said *wabi sabi* is "a bit like love." What I have discovered along the way is that actually *wabi sabi* is a lot like love. It is akin to loving appreciation—for beauty, for nature, for ourselves, for one another, and for life itself.

I hope you, too, have seen how *wabi sabi* can be a refreshing antidote to our fast-paced, consumption-driven world, and that it has encouraged you to slow down, reconnect with nature, and be gentler on yourself. I hope you have been inspired to simplify everything and concentrate on what really matters, finding happiness right where you are.

As we come to the end of our journey together, I have one final souvenir for you. Hold out your hands and imagine your gift. It is an *omamori* (お守り), an amulet to keep you safe as you journey forward. On the front is embroidered the character *sachi* (幸), for happiness.[2] On the back is written a gentle reminder:

You are perfectly imperfect,
just as you are.

後書き

ACKNOWLEDGMENTS

P ractically speaking, the wheels of this book were set in motion over steaming bowls of noodles at a rāmen bar in London, with my brilliant agent, Caroline Hardman of Hardman & Swainson. I am eternally grateful to Caroline for her unending enthusiasm for this project, and to her colleague Thérèse Coen for getting it into the hands of people all over the world, in many different languages. It is an absolute privilege to share my love of all things Japanese with so many people, and I hope this book inspires you to make your own visit to Japan.

I offer a deep bow to my marvelous editor, Anna Steadman, to Jillian Stewart, Anne Newman, Beth Wright, Aimee Kitson, Bekki Guyatt, and the rest of the fantastic team at Piatkus and Little, Brown, for bringing this book to life, getting it out into the world in such a beautiful way, and allowing me to do what I love and call it work. And I would like to say a special thank-you to my friend Hidetoshi Nakata for the beautiful foreword he shared in this book.

The truth is, I have been carrying this book inside me for the best part of two decades, and for that I am deeply grateful to my friends and surrogate families in Japan (the Itōs, the Adachis, and Hilary Frank), and my long-suffering teachers at the University of Durham, the University of Bath, and the Kyōto Institute of Culture and Language, as well as the many strangers who have shown me extraordinary kindness along the way.

I owe a huge debt of gratitude to Dr. Naomi Cross, Kaori Nishizawa, Hiroko Tamaki, and Bruce Hamana for their support in checking Japanese language and cultural references and historical facts, and for their incredible patience in the face of my endless questions. Any errors that slipped through the net are solely my responsibility.

This journey has been a treasure hunt. Every conversation held a clue. Throwaway comments led to particular books or poems or places. A friend of a friend's introduction to "someone you must meet" has led to unexpected insights and yet more introductions. It was quite daunting to head out on this journey truly not knowing where it would take me, but it has been worth the leap of faith.

Outside of the history books, cultural salons, shrines, temples, and forests, I found the real truth of *wabi sabi* in the hearts of people who showed me, without always telling me, what it can teach us. My particular thanks go to: Ai Matsuyama, Atsushi Hioki, Ayumi Nagata, Chikako Hosoya, Daisuke Sanada, Duncan Flett, Hiroko Tayama, Hiroshi Nagashima, Izumi Texidor Hirai, Kazuma Sugimoto, Kao Sōsa, Ken Igarashi, Kumiko Miyazaki, Kyōji Miura, Kyōko Adachi, Louie Miura, Louise Arai, Mai Nishiyama, Makiko Hastings, Master Hoshino, Matthew Claudel, Michiyuki Adachi, Mina Fujita, Mineyo Kanie, Nele Duprix, Norifumi Fujita, Noriko Hara, Pia Jane Bijkerk, Professor Peter Cheyne, Reishi Tayama, Saeko Tsukimi, Sara Kabariti, Sayaka Sanada, Seiko Mabuchi, Setsuko Sakae, Shigeyuki and Hiroko Shimizu, Shōji Maeda, Shōjirō Frank, Shūichi Haruyama, Reverend Takafumi Kawakami, Takashi Okuno, Takayuki Odajima, Dr. Teruaki Matsuzaki, Tetsuo Shimizu, Tim Romero, Tina Sakuragi, Tomi Matsuba, Toshinao Iwaki, Wataru Kataoka,

Yōko Kurisu, Yoshinao Kanie, Yukako Itō, Yumiko Sekine, and Yumiko Tanaka.

I am also grateful to the incredibly helpful staff of the Bodleian Japanese Library (University of Oxford), the SOAS Library (University of London), the Smithsonian Institute (Washington, D.C.), the Raku Museum, the Forestry and Fisheries Department of the Takashima city government, and the Elderly Welfare Department of the Nagoya city government.

Warm thanks go to the staff of Shunkō-in Temple, the House of Light, japan-experience.com, Mettricks, and the Arvon Foundation who gave me homes for writing. Particular thanks go to Emily, Jayne, and Marilyn for that first reading by the wood burner.

Huge thanks go to Lilla Rogers, Rachael Taylor, and Kelly Rae Roberts—the most generous and supportive business partners I could hope for. And to our team, without whom there would have been no time to write: Jitna Bhagani, Louise Gale, Vic Dickenson, Holly Wells, Kelly Crossley, Simon Brown, Rachael Hibbert, Mark Burgess, Liam Frost, Fiona Duffy, Rachel Kempton, Nichole Poinski. I also bow deeply to Jonathan Fields and Dr. Martin Shaw for their inspiring mentorship.

And to the thousands of people in my wonderful community at www.dowhatyouloveforlife.com and all the female entrepreneurs in our members' club, www.hellosoulhellobusiness.com, who have shared stories, challenges, and celebrations since we began the company almost a decade ago. You have my deepest respect for showing up, opening up, and trusting the journey.

There are never enough words to thank my parents for supporting my crazy idea to learn Japanese all those years ago (and all the other crazy ideas I have had since). I am also grateful to them and my parents-in-law, for the generous help that has made it possible to write two books while my children are still under five. *Otsukaresama deshita.*

And most of all, to Mr. K, for holding down the fort while I traveled and wrote, for learning Japanese, so you could speak to my friends, and for being the best life partner I could have ever hoped for. I have never met anyone with such an enormous heart, and sharing my life with you and our two gorgeous children is my greatest joy. To those daughters, Sienna and Maia, I cannot wait to share my love of Japan with you one day soon.

NOTES

注

Chapter 1:
Origins, characteristics, and relevance of *wabi sabi* today

1. There is no singular reference to *wabi sabi* in the 2018 edition of Japan's leading dictionary, *Kōjien*.

2. What we know as the written Japanese kanji characters originated in China. Nearly every one of the 1,850 standard characters in use today can be read in at least two different ways, with one reading derived from the original Chinese (known as *on'yomi*) and the other an indigenous Japanese reading (known as *kun'yomi*). Some characters have more than one of each reading. When two kanji are used together to create a word, the *on'yomi* is usually used. Rather confusingly, as an exception to this, our central concept of *wabi sabi* can be written as both 侘寂 and 侘び寂び. If you are interested in learning more about the fascinating world of kanji, I highly recommend *The Modern Reader's Japanese-English Character Dictionary* or *NTC's New Japanese-English Character Dictionary*.

3. The family name of Murata Shukō was Murata, but he is commonly known by the name of Shukō. This is often the case with the names of historical figures.

4. Okakura, *The Book of Tea,* p. 3.

5. From humble beginnings, Chōjirō pioneered the making of raku tea bowls and established the Raku family in the late sixteenth century, which has become the unique preserver of the raku-*yaki* pottery tradition. The current Raku Kichizaemon XV, a ceramic artist, is the fifteenth-generation head. Tea bowls fashioned by each generation can be seen at the Raku Museum in Kyōto (raku-yaki.or.jp/e/museum/index.html).

6. Nelson (ed.), *The Modern Reader's Japanese-English Character Dictionary*, p. 141.

7. Occasionally, 詫びる, a homophone of the verb *wabiru*, meaning "to apologize," is referenced in discussions related to the spirit of *wabi*, although the etymological connection is difficult to verify from reputable sources.

8. According to Japan's leading dictionary, *Kōjien, wabishii* means "a feeling of losing energy" or "feeling anxious or sad," but Japanese people commonly use *wabishii* to mean "wretched," "lonely," or "poor."

9. For further insight into the aesthetics of *wabi*, I recommend the excellent essay "The Wabi Aesthetic Through the Ages" by Haga Kōshirō, in Hume, *Japanese Aesthetics and Culture*, p. 275.

10. McKinney (trans.), *Essays in Idleness and Hōjōki*, p. 87.

11. Nelson (ed.), *The Modern Reader's Japanese English Character Dictionary*, p. 323. In the case of the character 寂, it has a *kun'yomi* reading of *sabi* and an *on'yomi* reading of *jaku* (meaning "tranquility"), as you will see in chapter 6. See note 2 above for more about *kun'yomi* and *on'yomi* readings in the Japanese language.

12. Nelson (ed.), *The Modern Reader's Japanese-English Character Dictionary*, p. 323. When read as *jaku*, the character 寂 means "tranquility" as explained in note 11, above.

13. Ibid.

14. Tanizaki, *In Praise of Shadows*, p. 19.

15. Matsuo Bashō, whose poetry is frequently cited as an example of literature with an air of *sabi*, lived the life of a *wabibito*—a person of *wabi*. Although not penniless, Bashō chose to wander long distances in nature, carrying with him only the bare minimum needed for survival. These journeys were the inspiration for his famous poetry.

16. Morigami, *Wabi sabi yūgen no kokoro*, p. 19.

17. Joyce, *A Portrait of the Artist as a Young Man*, p. 231.

Chapter 2:
Simplifying + beautifying

1. Source: Statistics Bureau, Ministry of Internal Affairs and Communications, government of Japan www.stat.go.jp/english /data/handbook/c0117.html.

2. Ibid.

3. According to the Tōkyō Metropolitan Government, the population of Tōkyō in 2015 was 13.491 million, around 11 percent of the national population. Source: www.metro.tokyo.jp/english/about /history/history03.html. Retrieved April 8, 2018.

4. A tatami mat is a Japanese flooring material, traditionally made from straw, often with brocade edging. Each mat is twice as long as it is wide. Tatami mats are used as a measure of room size in Japan (rather than imperial square feet or metric square meters). The area of one tatami mat is known as one *jō*. And it's not just inside the home—land is traditionally measured in *tsubo*, with one *tsubo* being the equivalent area of two tatami mats. In contemporary Japan, even people living in Western-style homes often have at least one Japanese-style room, known as a *washitsu*, with a tatami-matted floor.

5. Kanji are the adopted logographic Chinese characters that are used in the Japanese writing system, alongside the syllabaries *hiragana* and *katakana*.

6. You can find Makiko and her work online at makikohastings.com.

7. The word *maiko*, which translates to "dancing child," refers to an apprentice *geiko* (*geiko* being the name for a geisha from Kyōto). Geisha are women highly trained in traditional Japanese arts, including singing, dancing, and music, who have become a recognized symbol of Japan for many foreigners. *Maiko* often wear brightly colored, long-sleeved kimonos. Their accompanying obi (sash) is usually tied at their back and extends to their feet.

8. An obi is a sash worn with a kimono.

9. *Hagi-yaki* (萩焼), or "Hagi ware," is a type of Japanese pottery originating from the town of Hagi, in Yamaguchi Prefecture.

10. Yanagi, *The Unknown Craftsman*, p. 148.

11. Originally, *shibui* meant "astringent," such as the flavor of an under-ripe persimmon. Over the years, it has taken on an important aesthetic meaning and in 1960 was hailed by *House Beautiful* magazine as "the height of Japanese beauty" (see Gordon [ed.], *House Beautiful*, August 1960, USA edition).

12. Other important aesthetic principles include *miyabi* (refined elegance) and *suki* (originally "refinement with a hint of eccentricity, idiosyncrasy, or irregularity").

13. The Heian period in Japanese history (794–1185) "saw the full assimilation of Chinese culture and the flowering of an elegant courtly culture." Source: *The Kōdansha Bilingual Encyclopedia of Japan*, p. 100.

14. Source: "What Is Beauty? Can You Afford Any of It?" by Elizabeth Gordon, in Gordon (ed.), *House Beautiful*, May 1958, USA edition.

15. For a more formal analysis of Japanese aesthetics, I recommend the 1998 essay "Japanese Aesthetics," in *Japanese Aesthetics and Culture: A Reader* (ed. Nancy G. Hume), by distinguished Japan scholar Donald Keene. With extensive reference to poet and essayist Yoshida Kenkō's *Tsurezuregusa* (*Essays in Idleness*), Keene selected four key themes to suggest the main features of Japanese aesthetic taste as it has evolved over time. These were: suggestion, irregularity, simplicity, and perishability. Elements of these are included in the themes I have suggested for the soulful simplification of your home, although the five themes I offer include contemporary design ideas and are intended to be applicable to any home, anywhere. Aside from this, in his 1982 work, *Zen and the Fine Arts*, the late philosopher Shin'ichi Hisamatsu summarized his own observations into seven characteristics of Zen aesthetics as follows: asymmetry, simplicity, austere sublimity or lofty dryness, naturalness, subtle profundity or deep reserve, freedom from attachment, tranquility. These have been back-translated into Japanese in various different ways, but the most common words used are: *fukinsei* (不均整), *kanso* (簡素), *shibumi* (渋味), *shizen* (自然), *yūgen* (幽玄), *datsuzoku* (脱俗), and *seijaku* (静寂) respectively.

16. Find out more about Fog Linen Work at foglinenwork.com.

17. Kondō, *The Life-Changing Magic of Tidying*, p. 49.

18. According to architect Matthew Claudel, *ma* (間), the Japanese word for "space," goes beyond the Western concept of physical space to refer to the natural distance between two or more things existing in a continuity, the natural pause or interval between two or more phenomena occurring continuously and the space delineated by posts and screens in traditional Japanese architecture. Source: Claudel, *Ma: Foundations for the Relationship of Space-Time in Japanese Architecture*, p. 3.

19. Lafcadio Hearn (1850–1904), born to a Greek mother and an Irish father, and also known as Koizumi Yakumo since his naturalization as a Japanese, was a writer and translator best known for his books that introduced Japan to the West.

20. Hearn, *Japan: An Attempt at Interpretation*, "Strangeness and Charm" chapter (no page number).

Chapter 3:
Living with nature

1. Source: https://dictionary.cambridge.org/dictionary/english /nature#dataset-cald4/. Retrieved March 31, 2018.

2. The definition is listed as 「あるがままのさま。」(*arugamama no sama*). Source: Shinmura (ed.), *Kōjien: Dai 5 han*, p. 1174.

3. This is the poem as I remember it from my youth, but I have been unable to find the source of this particular translation. To explore Matsuo Bashō's poetry, I highly recommend works by Donald Keene, Makoto Ueda, Nobuyuki Yuasa, or Jane Reichhold.

4. Sei (trans. McKinney), *The Pillow Book*, p. 3.

5. In Japanese, the same name can be written in various ways, using different kanji characters, just as there are various spellings of the same name in English, (e.g., Clare and Claire). Source: https:// st.benesse.ne.jp/ninshin/name/2017. Retrieved March 30, 2018.

6. Source: www.jref.com/articles/japanese-family-names.31. Retrieved March 30, 2018.

7. There is also a "rainy season" in Japan known as *tsuyu*, although this does not qualify as a formal season. It can be anywhere between May and July, depending on location.

8. The wonderful free app 72 Seasons updates every five days with information about the nature, food, and tradition particular to that time in the classical Japanese calendar. www.kurashikata .com/72seasons.

9. Deal, *Handbook to Life in Medieval and Early Modern Japan,* p. 43.

10. There are various translations for the names of each of the seventy-two microseasons. Some of my favorites (and those shared in this book) appear in Liza Dalby's wonderful memoir of the seasons, *East Wind Melts the Ice.* Dalby, *East Wind Melts the Ice,* p. 287.

11. Deal, *Handbook to Life in Medieval and Early Modern Japan,* p. 190.

12. Yamakage, *The Essence of Shinto*, p. 29.

13. Ono, *Shinto*, p. 97.

14. See http://yamabushido.jp/ for further information about Yamabushi training.

15. Source: www.ncbi.nlm.nih.gov/pmc/articles/PMC4997467. Retrieved March 20, 2018.

16. Source: www.ncbi.nlm.nih.gov/pubmed/20074458. Retrieved March 20, 2018.

17. Miyazaki, *Shinrin-yoku*, p. 11.

18. Miyazaki, *Shinrin-yoku*, p. 23.

19. Doi, *The Anatomy of Self,* p. 159.

20. The Meiji Restoration in 1868 restored practical imperial rule to Japan. Even though there had been ruling emperors before this, their practical powers and influence were limited. The restoration brought to an end a 250-year period known as *sakoku,* the foreign-relations policy that saw Japan almost entirely closed off to foreign influence. This led to huge changes in Japan's political and social structure, and a race to catch up with Western technology.

Chapter 4:
Acceptance + letting go

1. As told to me by Reverend Takafumi Kawakami, deputy head priest of the Shunkō-in Temple in Kyōto.
2. Ostaseski, *The Five Invitations*, p. 116.

Chapter 5:
Reframing failure

1. The full interview can be heard at www.disruptingjapan.com /the-myth-of-the-sucessful-startup-failure-hiroshi-nagashima.
2. You can find out more about the House of Light at www .hikarinoyakata.com.
3. *Sukiya-zukuri* or "*sukiya* style" is a type of Japanese residential architectural style. Its origins lie in tearoom architecture, and it has come to indicate a style of designing that embodies refined, well-cultivated taste. It is characterized by the use of natural materials based on teahouse aesthetics.
4. For further architectural details, see Taschen, *Living in Japan*, p. 88.

Chapter 6:
Nurturing relationships

1. The four principles of the tea ceremony, *wa kei sei jaku* (和敬清寂), harmony, respect, purity, and tranquility, were handed down from Sen no Rikyū, the "father of tea." There are three Sen houses/families of tea in Japan, known as Urasenke, Omotesenke, and Mushakōjinosenke. These three separate family lines were established by the three sons of Sen no Rikyū's grandson Sen Sōtan. Three main words are used in Japanese for what we call the tea ceremony in English. *Chanoyu* (茶の湯), literally "hot water for tea," is the word used to refer to the act of making and serving tea. *Sadō* and *chadō* are alternative readings for 茶道, "the way of tea." According to tea instructor Bruce Hamana of the Urasenke school, knowing the technical elements of *chanoyu* alone does not make the

tea ceremony a way of understanding ourselves and the world. He told me: "Constant discipline and consideration of our guests can help us go beyond our attachment to material things." He believes this spiritual element is the essence of "the way of tea," *sadō* or *chadō*.

2. Source: www.urasenke.org/characters/index.html. Retrieved January 15, 2018.

3. Reverend Kawakami also explained the second meaning of "no self" in Buddhism, as referring to "the way that our self does not have ultimate control over our mind or body." He shared meditation as an example, where we focus on our breathing but a moment later our mind starts wandering. In much the same way, he said this "no self" means we cannot stop ourselves from getting old.

4. Source: "Loneliness Connects Us: Young People Exploring and Experiencing Loneliness and Friendship," 2018 report from Manchester Metropolitan University and 42nd Street, supported by the Coop Foundation. https://mcrmetropolis.uk/wp-content /uploads/Loneliness-Connects-Us.pdf. Retrieved March 20, 2018.

5. Source: https://reliefweb.int/report/world/global-peace-index -2017. Retrieved March 22, 2018. Japan was in the top ten in the 2017 report (joint 10th), 2015 report (8th), and 2013 report (6th). Retrieved March 22, 2018.

6. Source: www.telegraph.co.uk/travel/lists/most-peaceful -countries/japan. Retrieved March 22, 2018.

7. *Pachinko* is a kind of pinball arcade game popular in Japan. Each machine fires hundreds of small steel balls in multiple directions, so the collective sound inside an arcade can be deafening, like an incessant crashing and banging of pans.

Chapter 7:
Enjoying the career journey

1. Iwami Ginzan Silver Mine is on the UNESCO World Heritage List (Source: https://whc.unesco.org/en/list/1246. Retrieved April 9, 2018), and Ōmori-chō is involved in a UNESCO Education for Sustainable Development (ESD) project (Source: www.unesco.org/new/en/media-services/single-view/news/

big_experiment_in_sustainable_development_education
_transfor. Retrieved April 9, 2018).

2. In much the same way as the Slow Food movement founded by Carlo Petroni is based on a philosophy of nutritious and tasty food, sustainably and locally grown "slow clothing" is a way of thinking about the clothes we buy and wear to ensure they bring meaning, value, and joy to every day, while minimizing their negative impact in terms of environmental and social challenges.

3. Gungendō is the lifestyle brand of the Iwami-Ginzan Lifestyle Research Institute, which Tomi cofounded with her husband, Daikichi. Find out more at www.gungendo.co.jp.

4. See inside at www.kurasuyado.jp/takyo-abeke.

5. De Mente, *NTC's Dictionary of Japan's Business Code Words,* p. 196.

6. Originally called *jōjutsu* (杖術), the name of this martial art changed to *jōdō* (杖道) "the way of the staff" in 1940. It was devised by master swordsman Gonnosuke Katsukichi in the early 1600s. Source: www.britishkendoassociation.com/jodo. Retrieved April 11, 2018.

7. Sen, *Nihonjin no kokoro, tsutaemasu,* p. 88.

8. Gratton and Scott's, *The 100-Year Life* provides an excellent summary of the latest evidence on this topic.

9. Source: *Workforce of the future: the competing forces shaping 2030* (PwC report). Available from https://www.pwc.com/gx/en /services/people-organisation/workforce-of-the-future/workforce -of-the-future-the-competing-forces-shaping-2030-pwc.pdf. Retrieved April 2, 2018.

10. Ibid.

11. A *furoshiki* is a type of cloth traditionally used to wrap gifts, food, or other goods.

12. 日々是好日 can also be read as *hibi kore kōjitsu.*

Chapter 8: Cherishing the moments

1. Source: UNDP http://hdr.undp.org/en/69206. Retrieved April 6, 2018.

2. Source: Ministry of Health, Labour and Welfare, government of

Japan, www.mhlw.go.jp/file/04-Houdouhappyou-12304250
-Roukenkyoku-Koureishashienka/0000177627.pdf. Retrieved
April 6, 2018.

3. Source: Ministry of Health, Labour and Welfare, government of
Japan, www.mhlw.go.jp/toukei/saikin/hw/life/ckts10/dl/02.pdf.
Retrieved April 6, 2018.

4. Source: http://president.jp/articles/-/15634. Retrieved
April 6, 2018.

5. Source: Nagano Prefectural Government www.pref.nagano
.lg.jp/kenko-fukushi/kenko/kenko/documents/saisyueiyaku.pdf.
Retrieved April 6, 2018.

6. Source: www.reuters.com/brandfeatures/venture-capital
/article?id=11480. Retrieved February 26, 2018.

7. Source: WHO 2017 World Malaria Report, www.who.int/malaria
/publications/world-malaria-report-2017/report/en. Retrieved
February 18, 2018.

8. As designated by the *Shūkan Gendai* weekly magazine, December 9,
2017, edition.

9. For a step-by-step guide to getting your life organized, try my
online course *How to be Happy (Calm, Organized + Focused)*. Details
at www.dowhatyouloveforlife.com.

Afterword:
Tying it all together

1. Raku (trans. Faulkner and Andō), *Chawanya*, p. 105.
2. The word most commonly used for happiness in Japan is *shiawase*,
written 幸せ. However, when it is shown as a single character, 幸,
for example on lucky charms at temples, it is read as *sachi*.

日本を旅する

NOTES ON
VISITING JAPAN

f this book has inspired you to visit Japan, I am thrilled! Here are a few thoughts to help you prepare. For my up-to-date personal recommendations of places to go and things to do and see, visit www.bethkempton.com/japan.

And be sure to tag me @bethkempton on Instagram, so I can get a peek at your adventures.

How to travel in Japan

- Go with an open mind and an open heart.
- Learn a few words of Japanese before you go—even a single greeting goes a long way, and recognizing a few simple characters can give you confidence.
- Practice using chopsticks.
- Respect local customs: remove your shoes before going indoors, don't blow your nose in public, don't drop litter, don't tip, don't eat in the street.
- If you take a bath in a public *sento* or *onsen*, wash *before* you get in the bath.
- Talk to local people whenever you can.
- Take small gifts in case you have the chance to visit someone's home.
- Generally Japan is a quiet place. Keep the noise down, especially in temples, shrines, and gardens.
- Smile, you're having an adventure!

Tips on planning

It can be tempting to just go to the places you have heard of, but much magic and mystery lie off the beaten track. If you aren't sure where to start planning your journey, try picking a theme and go from there. Here are a few ideas:

Start with an *onsen*

There are thousands of *onsen* (hot springs) all over Japan, many of them in remote towns and villages, some on mountainsides, others by the ocean. All offer an authentic experience of Japanese life, a delight for your body and a soothing experience for your mind. You'll also likely experience warm hospitality and amazing food. *Ryokan* are a wonderful indulgence if your budget can accommodate it. Otherwise, try staying in a local inn (*minshuku*) or Airbnb and just go to the hot spring as a day visitor, often for just a few hundred yen. To begin your search, type *onsen*, plus the area of Japan you'd like to visit into Google, click on "Images," and take it from there.

Go for the food

Every prefecture, city, and town in Japan is famous for something, very often a particular kind of food. Going on a foodie tour of the country can be a wonderful way to explore outside the regular routes and discover all sorts of culinary delights. Why not challenge yourself to find the best rāmen or to sample some particular type of mountain vegetable?

Discover traditional crafts

Go in search of a craft you are interested in. Some of the best potteries in the country are located in beautiful rural towns and villages and can make a great base for hiking or otherwise enjoying the countryside.

Go skiing/snowboarding
Japan has some of the best snow in the world, with slopes that are often much emptier than their European counterparts. Plus, they serve Japanese curry on the slopes, and offer hot springs and snow festivals. Try Nagano, Hokkaidō, or Zao (between Yamagata and Sendai).

Rent a house
Staying in a traditional house, or doing a homestay with a family, can be a wonderful experience. Instead of rushing from place to place, consider staying for a while in one place, getting to know the local area, and imagining yourself living there.

Have a magical mystery tour
Get yourself a JR Pass (a great value rail pass) before you go, then close your eyes, put your finger on the rail map, and go there. See what you find!

Useful websites

www.bethkempton.com/japan for my free Japan guides
www.jnto.go.jp/eng website of the Japan National Tourism
    Organization
www.japan-guide.com for planning your trip
www.hyperdia.com or the Hyperdia app for train timetables
www.rometorio.com for planning journeys between any
    two places
http://willerexpress.com/en for cheap long-distance buses

www.co-ba.net for coworking spaces

www.japan-experience.com for lovely Japanese homes to rent

www.airbnb.com for homes and apartments to rent

nakata.net/rnp for Hidetoshi Nakata's diary of the seven years
he spent traveling throughout Japan. This phenomenal
resource introduces some of the most inspiring artisans,
sake breweries, handcrafted products, and beautiful places
to stay, all across the country.

www.jisho.org for Japanese-English translation. This site allows
you to draw in kanji characters.

waygoapp.com for menu translation

jpninfo.com for a Japan visitor guide written by Japanese people

taiken.co for up-to-date visitor information

www.tofugu.com for a brilliant blog about all things Japanese

www.japan-talk.com for all sorts of mini travel guides

www.japantimes.co.jp, japantoday.com, mainichi.jp/english for
daily news

jetprogramme.org for the Japan Exchange and Teaching
Programme, if you fancy a career break or a new challenge

en.air-j.info for an online database of artist-in-residence
opportunities in Japan

Useful apps

For travel:
Hyperdia
Navitime
Maps with Me
Tokoyo Subway Navigation
Japan Taxi

For food:
Gurunavi

For language:
Imiwa
Yomiwa

Others:
Yurekuru Call (for earthquake info)
Line (for instant messaging)
XE Currency Converter
72 Seasons

参考文献

BIBLIOGRAPHY

English-language sources

Abe, Hajime. *The View of Nature in Japanese Literature*. Chiba: Tōyō Gakuen University Faculty of Humanities, 2011.

Anesaki, Masaharu. *Art, Life & Nature in Japan*. Rutland, Vermont: Tuttle, 1964.

Bailly, Sandrine. *Japan: Season by Season*. New York: Abrams, 2009.

Bellah, Robert N. *Imagining Japan: The Japanese Tradition and Its Modern Interpretation*. Berkeley: University of California Press, 2003.

Castile, Rand. *The Way of Tea*. New York: Weatherill, 1971.

Channell, Sōei Randy. *The Book of Chanoyu*. Tōkyō: Tankōsha, 2016.

Chiba, Fumiko. *Kakeibo: The Japanese Art of Saving Money*. London: Penguin, 2017.

Claudel, Matthew. *Ma: Foundations for the Relationship of Space-Time to Japanese Architecture, Exhibition Catalogue*. New Haven: University of Yale, MA thesis, 2012.

Dalby, Liza. *East Wind Melts the Ice: A Memoir Through the Seasons*. London: Chatto & Windus, 2007.

Davies, Roger J. *Japanese Culture: The Religious and Philosophical Foundations*. Rutland, Vermont: Tuttle, 2016.

Davies, Roger J., and Ikeno Osamu, eds., *The Japanese Mind: Understanding Contemporary Japanese Culture.* Rutland, Vermont: Tuttle, 2002.

De Mente, Boye Lafayette. *NTC's Dictionary of Japan's Business Code Words.* London: McGraw-Hill, 1997.

—. *NTC's Dictionary of Japan's Cultural Code Words.* London: McGraw-Hill, 1996.

Deal, William E. *Handbook to Life in Medieval and Early Modern Japan.* Oxford: Oxford University Press, 2007.

Doi, Takeo. *The Anatomy of Dependence.* Tōkyō: Kōdansha, 1973.

—. *The Anatomy of Self: Individual Versus Society.* Tōkyō: Kōdansha, 1985.

Freeman, Michael. *Mindful Design of Japan: 40 Modern Tea-Ceremony Rooms.* London: Eight Books, 2007.

Gordon, Elizabeth, ed., *House Beautiful* (May 1958, August 1960, and September 1960 USA editions)

Gratton, Lynda, and Scott Andrew. *The 100-Year Life: Living and Working in an Age of Longevity.* London: Bloomsbury, 2017.

Halpern, Jack, ed., *NTC's New Japanese-English Character Dictionary.* London: McGraw-Hill Contemporary, 1994.

Hearn, Lafcadio. *Gleanings in Buddha-Fields: Studies of Hand and Soul in the Far East.* London: Cape, 1927.

—. *Japan: An Attempt at Interpretation.* New York: Macmillan, 1904.

Hendry, Joy. *Wrapping Culture: Politeness, Presentation and Power in Japan and Other Countries.* Oxford: Clarendon Press, 1993.

Hisamatsu, Shin'ichi. *Zen and the Fine Arts.* New York: Kōdansha, 1982.

Holthus, Barbara G., and Manzenreiter Wolfram. *Life Course,*

Happiness and Wellbeing in Japan. London: Routledge, 2017.

Hume, Nancy G., ed., *Japanese Aesthetics and Culture: A Reader*. New York: State University of New York Press, 1995.

Itō, Teiji. ed., *Wabi Sabi Suki: The Essence of Japanese Beauty*. Hiroshima: Mazda Motor Corporation, 1993.

Joycc, James. *A Portrait of the Artist as a Young Man*. London: Penguin Classics, 2000.

Juniper, Andrew. *Wabi Sabi: The Japanese Art of Impermanence*. Rutland, Vermont: Tuttle, 2003.

Kawano, Satsuki, Glenda S. Roberts, and Susan Orpett Long. *Capturing Contemporary Japan: Differentiation and Uncertainty*. Honolulu: University of Hawai'i Press, 2014.

Kenkō and Chōmei. *Essays in Idleness and Hōjōki*. Translated by Meredith McKinney. London: Penguin Classics, 2013.

Kerr, Alex. *Another Kyoto*. Tōkyō: Sekai Bunka Publishing, 2016.

—. *Lost Japan*. London: Penguin, 2015.

Kōdansha International, eds. *The Kodansha Bilingual Encyclopedia of Japan*. Tōkyō: Kōdansha, 1998.

Kondō, Marie. *The Life-Changing Magic of Tidying: A Simple Effective Way to Banish Clutter Forever*. London: Vermillion, 2014.

Landis, Barnhill David. *Moments, Season, and Mysticism: The Complexity of Time in Japanese Haiku*. Transcript of speech at ASLE conference at Wofford College, Spartanburg, SC, 2007, available at www.uwosh.edu/facstaff/barnhill /es-244-basho/moments.pdf. Accessed April 12, 2018.

MacDonald, Deanna. *Eco Living Japan*. Rutland, Vermont: Tuttle, 2015.

Matsuo, Bashō. *Basho: The Complete Haiku*. Translated by Jane Reichhold. New York: Kōdansha, 2008.

—. *The Narrow Road to the Deep North and Other Travel Sketches*. Translated by Nobuyuki Yuasa. London: Penguin Classics, 1966.

Miner, Earl. *An Introduction to Japanese Court Poetry*. Stanford: Stanford University Press, 1968.

Miyazaki, Yoshifumi. *Shinrin-yoku: The Japanese Way of Forest Bathing for Health and Relaxation*. London: Aster, 2018.

Moeran, Brian. *Language and Popular Culture in Japan*. Manchester: Manchester University Press, 1989.

Mogi, Ken. *The Little Book of Ikigai*. London: Quercus, 2017.

Nelson, Andrew N., ed. *The Modern Reader's Japanese-English Character Dictionary*. Rutland, Vermont: Tuttle, 1993.

Okakura, Kakuzo. *The Book of Tea*. London: Penguin Random House, 2016.

Ono, Sokyō. *Shinto: The Kami Way*. Rutland, Vermont: Tuttle, 1962.

Ostaseski, Frank. *The Five Invitations: Discovering What Death Can Teach Us About Living Fully*. London: Bluebird, 2017.

Pilling, David. *Bending Adversity: Japan and the Art of Survival*. London: Penguin, 2014.

Reynolds, David K. *The Quiet Therapies: Japanese Pathways to Personal Growth*. Honolulu: University of Hawai'i Press, 1980.

Raku, Kichizaemon. *Chawanya*. Translated by Rupert Faulkner and Kyōko Andō. Tōkyō: Tankōsha, 2012.

Richie, Donald. *A Tractate on Japanese Aesthetics*. Berkeley: Stone Bridge Press, 2007.

Rousemaniere, Nicole, ed., *Crafting Beauty in Modern Japan*. London: The British Museum Press, 2007.

Saitō, Yuriko. *Aesthetics of the Familiar: Everyday Life and World-Making*. Oxford: Oxford University Press, 2017.

Satsuka, Shiho. *Nature in Translation*. Durham: Duke University Press, 2015.

Sei, Shōnagon. *The Pillow Book*. Translated by Meredith McKinney. London: Penguin Classics, 2006.

Stevens, John. *Three Zen Masters: Ikkyū, Hakuin, Ryōkan*. New York: Kōdansha, 1993.

Suzuki, Daisetz T. *Zen and Japanese Culture*. Princeton: Princeton University Press, 2010.

Takishita, Yoshihiro. *Japanese Country Style*. Tōkyō: Kōdansha, 2002.

Tanahashi, Kazuaki. *Sky Above, Great Wind: The Life and Poetry of Zen Master Ryōkan*. Boston: Shambhala, 2012.

Tanaka, Sen'ō, and Tanaka Sendō. *The Tea Ceremony*. Tōkyō: Kōdansha, 1998.

Tanizaki, Jun'ichirō. *In Praise of Shadows*. London: Vintage, 2001.

Taschen, Angelika, ed., *Living in Japan*. Cologne: Taschen, 2006.

Ueda, Makoto. *Literary and Art Theories in Japan*. Ann Arbor: University of Michigan, 1991.

Van Koesveld, Robert. *Geiko and Maiko of Kyoto*. Sydney: Presence Publishing, 2015.

Williams, Florence. *The Nature Fix: Why Nature Makes Us Happier, Healthier and More Creative*. New York: Norton, 2018.

Yamada, Shōji. *Shots in the Dark: Japan, Zen and the West*. Chicago: University of Chicago Press, 2009.

Yamakage, Motohisa. *The Essence of Shinto: Japan's Spiritual Heart*. New York: Kōdansha, 2006.

Yamakuse, Yōji. *Japaneseness: A Guide to Values and Virtues*. Berkeley: Stone Bridge Press, 2016.

—. *Soul of Japan: The Visible Essence.* Tōkyō: IBC
    Publishing, 2012.
Yanagi, Sōetsu. *The Unknown Craftsman: A Japanese Insight into
    Beauty.* Tōkyō: Kōdansha, 1972.
Yokota, Nanrei. *Insights into Living: The Sayings of Zen Master
    Nanrei Yokota.* Tōkyō: Interbooks, 2016.

Japanese-language sources

Arikawa, Mayumi. *Nichijyō o, kokochiyoku.* Tōkyō: PHP, 2012.
Hayashi, Atsumu. *Tadashii kakei kanri* Tōkyō: Wave, 2014.
Hibi, Sadao, and Kazuya Takaoka. *Nihon no mado.* Tōkyō: Pie
    Books, 2010.
Hirai, Kazumi. *Kisetsu o tanoshimu riisuzukuri.* Tōkyō:
    Kawade, 2012.
Jingukan, ed., *Kurashi no shikitari jyūnikagetsu.* Tōkyō:
    Jingukan, 2014.
Korona, Bukkusu. *Washi no aru kurashi.* Tōkyō:
    Heibonsha, 2000.
Kunieda, Yasue. *Rinen to kurasu.* Tōkyō: Jakometei
    Shuppan, 2001.
Matsuba, Tomi. *Gungendō no ne no aru kurashi.* Tōkyō: Ie no
    Hikari Kyōkai, 2009.
Mori, Mayumi. *Kigyō wa sankan kara.* Tōkyō: Basilico, 2009.
Morigami, Shōyō. *Wabi sabi yūgen no kokoro: Seiyō tetsugaku o
    koeru jyōi ishiki.* Tōkyō: Sakuranohana Shuppan, 2015.
Natsui, Itsuki. *Utsukushiki, kisetsu to nihongo.* Tōkyō: Wani
    Books, 2015.
Okumura, Kumi. *Hibi, sensu o migaku kurashikata.* Tōkyō: Wani
    Books, 2007.

Rari, Yoshio. *Flower Book*. Tōkyō: Rikuyosha, 2005.

Sekai, Bunkasha Mook. *Wafū interia ga kimochi ii*. Tōkyō: Sekai Bunkasha, 2001.

Sekine, Yumiko. *Rinen wāku*. Tōkyō: Bunka Shuppankyoku, 2005.

Sen, Genshitsu. *Nihon no kokoro, tsutaemasu*. Tōkyō: Gentōsha, 2016.

Shinmura, Izuru, ed., *Kōjien: Dai 5 han*. Tōkyō: Iwanami Shoten, 1998.

—, ed., *Kōjien: Dai 7 han*. Tōkyō: Iwanami Shoten, 2018.

Shufu no Tomo, ed., *Shinrinyoku no mori hyaku sen*. Tōkyō, Shufu no Tomo, 2010.

Shufu to Seikatsu sha, ed., *Tegami no aru kurashi kokoro yutaka na*. Tōkyō: Shufu to Seikatsu sha, 2008.

Suzuki, Sadami, et al. *Wabi sabi yūgen: Nihonteki naru mono e no dōtei*. Tōkyō: Suiseisha, 2006.

Taki, Seiko. *Zakka no yukue* Tōkyō: Shufu no Tomo, 2001.

Uchida, Shigeru. *Interia to nihonjin*. Tōkyō: Shobunsha, 2000.

X-Knowledge. *Chiisana ie de tanoshimu sutairu no aru kurashi*. Tōkyō: X-Knowledge, 2015.

Yazaki, Junko. *Dezain to monozukuri no suteki na oshigoto*. Tōkyō: Bug News Network, 2009.

Yoshio, Akioka. *Shinwafū no susume*. Tōkyō: Kosei Shuppan, 1989.

Yuki, Anna. *Jibun o itawaru kurashigoto*. Tōkyō: Shufu to Seikatsu sha, 2017.

Yumioka, Katsumi. *Kimono to nihon no iro*. Tōkyō: Pie Books, 2005.

Index